KV-510-400

THE FUNCTIONS OF SLEEP

ACADEMIC PRESS RAPID MANUSCRIPT REPRODUCTION

*The proceedings of a symposium
held in Mexico City in August 1977.*

1340.

STIRLING UNIVERSITY LIBRARY

BOOK NUMBER   VOL COPY

0 9 5 6 0 6 — 1 1   WITHDRAWN

Stirling University Library (01786) 467220

09560611

date

STIRLING UNIVERSITY LIBRARY

BOOK LOAN

Please RETURN or RENEW it no later
than the last date shown below

29 NOV 1998 CANCELLED	2 5 MAY 2001	
2 8 MAY 1999 CANCELLED	2 5 MAY 2001	
	2 0 SEP 2002	
17 DEC 1999 CANCELLED		
2 6 MAY 2000		
2 6 MAY 2000		

B
8·53
DRU

THE FUNCTIONS OF SLEEP

WITHDRAWN

STIRLING UNIVERSITY LIBRARY

edited by

René Drucker-Colín

Departamento de Biología Experimental
Instituto de Biología
Universidad Nacional Autónoma de México
México, D.F., México

Mario Shkurovich

Servicio de Neurofisiología Clínica
Hospital del Niño, DIF
México, D.F., México

M. B. Sterman

V.A. Hospital
Sepulveda, California
and
Department of Anatomy
UCLA School of Medicine
Los Angeles, California

3/80

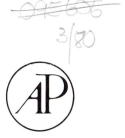

ACADEMIC PRESS   *New York   San Francisco   London*   **1979**
A Subsidiary of Harcourt Brace Jovanovich, Publishers

COPYRIGHT © 1979, BY ACADEMIC PRESS, INC.
ALL RIGHTS RESERVED.
NO PART OF THIS PUBLICATION MAY BE REPRODUCED OR
TRANSMITTED IN ANY FORM OR BY ANY MEANS, ELECTRONIC
OR MECHANICAL, INCLUDING PHOTOCOPY, RECORDING, OR ANY
INFORMATION STORAGE AND RETRIEVAL SYSTEM, WITHOUT
PERMISSION IN WRITING FROM THE PUBLISHER.

ACADEMIC PRESS, INC.
111 Fifth Avenue, New York, New York 10003

United Kingdom Edition published by
ACADEMIC PRESS, INC. (LONDON) LTD.
24/28 Oval Road, London NW1 7DX

Library of Congress Cataloging in Publication Data
Main entry under title:

The Functions of sleep.

Proceedings of a symposium sponsored by
Hospital del niño and Universidad Nacional
Autonoma de Mexico, Instituto de Biología,
Mexico, August 17-19, 1977.
1. Sleep—Physiological aspects—Congresses.
2. Sleep disorders—Congresses. I. Drucker-Colin,
René Raúl. II. Shkurovich, Mario. III. Sterman,
Barry M. IV. Mérida, Mexico. Hospital del niño.
V. Mexico (City). Universidad Nacional.
Instituto de Biologiá. [DNLM: 1. Sleep—
Physiology—Congresses. WL108 D794f 1977]
QP425.F86   612'.821   78-25669
ISBN O-12-222340-3

PRINTED IN THE UNITED STATES OF AMERICA

79 80 81 82 83 84   9 8 7 6 5 4 3 2 1

CONTENTS

CONTRIBUTORS   vii
PREFACE   ix
ACKNOWLEDGMENTS   xi

The Function of Sleep: Methodological Issues   1
Allan Rechtschaffen

Theories of Sleep Functions and Some Clinical Implications   19
Wilse B. Webb

Reticular Formation Activity and REM Sleep   37
Jerome M. Siegel

Sleep and Epilepsy: An Experimental Study   73
Marcos Velasco, Francisco Velasco, and Francisco Estrada-Villanueva

**Protein Molecules and the Regulation of REM Sleep: Possible Implications
for Function**   99
René Drucker-Colín

Growth Hormone Secretion Related to the Sleep and Waking Rhythm   113
Yasuro Takahashi

Neuropharmacologic and Neuroendocrine Interrelations of Human Sleep   147
H. Solis, A. Fernández-Guardiola, and C. Valverde - R.

Ontogenetic and Clinical Studies of Sleep State Organization and Dissociation 171
Dennis J. McGinty

Ontogeny of Sleep: Implications for Function   207
M. B. Sterman

A Motivational Function of REM Sleep   233
Gerald W. Vogel

What Can Insomniacs Teach Us About the Functions of Sleep?   251
Peter Hauri

The Relevance of Sleep Pathologies to the Function of Sleep   273
William C. Dement

Sleep, Brain State, and Memory   295
James L. McGaugh, Robert A. Jensen, and Joe L. Martinez, Jr.

CONTRIBUTORS

Numbers in parentheses indicate pages on which authors' contributions begin.

WILLIAM C. DEMENT *(273), Sleep Research Center, Stanford University School of Medicine, Stanford, California.*

RENÉ DRUCKER-COLÍN *(99), Departamento de Biologia Experimental, Instituto de Biologia, Universidad Nacional Autónoma de México, México, D. F., México.*

FRANCISCO ESTRADA-VILLANUEVA *(73), Division de Neurofisiología, Departamento de Investigación Cientifica, Centro Medico Nacional, IMSS, México, D. F., México*

AUGUSTO FERNANDEZ-GUARDIOLA *(147), Unidad de Investigaciones Cerebrales, Instituto Nacional de Neurologia, México, D. F., México.*

PETER HAURI *(251), Department of Psychiatry, Dartmouth Medical School, Hanover, New Hampshire.*

ROBERT A. JENSEN *(295), Department of Psychobiology, University of California, Irvine, California.*

JAMES L. McGAUGH *(295), Department of Psychobiology, University of California, Irvine, California.*

DENNIS J. McGINTY *(171), Veterans Administration Hospital, Sepulveda, California*

JOE L. MARTINEZ, JR. *(295), Department of Psychobiology, University of California, Irvine, California.*

ALLAN RECHTSCHAFFEN *(1), Sleep Laboratory, University of Chicago, Chicago, Illinois*

JEROME M. SIEGEL *(37), Neurophysiology Research, Veterans Administration Hospital, Sepulveda, California, and Brain Research Institute, University of California, Los Angeles, California.*

HUGO SOLIS *(147), Unidad de Investigaciones Cerebrales, Instituto Nacional de Neurología, México, D. F., México.*

M. B. STERMAN *(207), Veterans Administration Hospital, Sepulveda, California and UCLA School of Medicine, Los Angeles, California.*

YASURO TAKAHASHI *(113), Department of Psychology, Tokyo Metropolitan Institute for Neuroscience, Fuchu City, Tokyo, Japan.*

CARLOS VALVERDE-R. *(147), Departamento de Medicina Nuclear y Clinica de Tiroides, Instituto Nacional de la Nutrición, México, D. F., México.*

FRANCISCO VELASCO *(73), Division de Neurofisiologia, Departamento de Investigación Cientifica, Centro Medico Nacional IMSS, México, D. F., México.*

MARCOS VELASCO *(73), Division de Neurofisiología, Departamento de Investigación Cientifica, Centro Medico Nacional IMSS, México, D. F., México.*

GERALD W. VOGEL *(233), Emory University School of Medicine, Sleep Laboratory, Georgia Mental Health Institute, Atlanta, Georgia.*

WILSE B. WEBB *(19), Department of Psychology, University of Florida, Gainsville, Florida.*

PREFACE

Man has always been intrigued with the process of sleep. When technical means became available to explore this process scientifically, a systematic search for its functions was begun. In the context of evolutionary biology, sleep must contribute to survival and fitness and promote adaptation to environment and reproduction. Scientists and others assumed that sleep functioned to reverse the "fatigue" of sleeplessness, and attempted to define more precisely how fatigue affected the brain and body and how sleep reversed these effects. That search, however, disclosed a surprising fact. No matter what aspect of physiology or behavior was examined, its characteristics were significantly altered as a function of sleep states. While physiologists and later biochemists explored the basic dynamics exposed by these findings, clinicians focused on the psychological and medical implications of such alterations.

The search for function, however, was not entirely abandoned. A major effort was directed to the study of the effects of prolonged sleep deprivation. Another surprise was in store. Extended periods of enforced wakefulness did not appear to produce significant psychological or physical consequences other than sleepiness. While it was difficult to confirm absolute sleep deprivation in these studies, such findings threw doubt on the historically popular notion of sleep as an essential mechanism for reversal of some physiological substrate of fatigue.

The lack of focus on the question of the functions of sleep and the obvious absence of a simplistic answer to this question led us to organize a symposium on the topic. Our objective was to bring together an interdisciplinary group of productive investigators in the field of sleep research whose contributions, past and present, qualified them as spokesmen on this difficult issue. The meeting was held in August 1977 at Mexico City. This text is an outgrowth of that symposium. The papers presented address the question of the functions of sleep from a wide variety of perspectives, examining the developmental, neurophysiological, metabolic, behavioral, and clinical correlates of normal and disturbed sleep. Additionally, basic strategies and subtle pitfalls in the study of sleep functions are outlined in an unusually comprehensive methodological discussion.

Judging from the diversity of views expressed, it is clear that at least two positions must be considered. Either we still have failed to grasp the true functional significance of sleep or, in fact, sleep serves many adaptive purposes. Arguments presented in these pages appear to favor the latter position. Certainly, many important and perhaps fundamental points of view concerning the functions of sleep are not represented here. For this we apologize, both to their advocates and to the reader. However, what has been accomplished is a collection of contributions that focus on this question and depict the state-of-the-art in our quest for its answer. It is hoped that this compendium will facilitate further inquiry into this fundamental area of sleep research and discourage a narrow conceptualization of its boundaries.

ACKNOWLEDGMENTS

This symposium was supported by the Hospital del Niño, DIF and by the Universidad Nacional Autónoma de México. We wish to express our gratitude to Rosalia Zertuche de Drucker for spending countless hours in the never ending details necessary for preparing the manuscript. Above all, we are grateful to her for giving to this book with her good disposition an incredible amount of patience and attention.

THE FUNCTION OF SLEEP: METHODOLOGICAL ISSUES

ALLAN RECHTSCHAFFEN

Sleep Laboratory
University of Chicago
Chicago, Illinois

All of us who work on the function of sleep are fortunate to have such a virgin frontier as a challenge. The functional significance of most major biological systems such as respiration, circulation, and metabolism is largely understood, but we do not know why so much of our own lives, the lives of all mammals and, very likely, submammalian species as well, should be captured by sleep. The possible significance of the question almost exceeds imagination. When the layman asks why we study the function of sleep, we usually give practical answers, such as the possibility of learning how to fulfill the function more efficiently. However, the function of sleep might have a much deeper significance which extends across a large range of biological phenomena. For example, sleep might permit periodic readjustments of several biological systems or parts of a system to optimal relationships with each other; such readjustments might be difficult during wakefulness when more vigorous interaction with the environment creates differential demands on different components. Sleep function may have unsuspected implications for health and disease. Now we prescribe sleep like a folk remedy, but in spite of the age old admonition for the sick person to get plenty of sleep, I do not know of a single, well controlled study which demonstrates that sleep ever helped anyone get over any malady--except for lack of sleep. Some day we may be able to prescribe sleep for specific disorders because we know specifically what it does. Our current speculations about the function of sleep may turn out to be petty approximations of a huge significance that we will not really appreciate until we are part way toward the answer.

Copyright © 1979 by Academic Press, Inc.
All rights of reproduction in any form reserved.
ISBN 0-12-222340-3

Perhaps I do my colleagues an injustice. Some of them have offered theories of sleep function which may be prophetic visions of the truth. But if they are, these prophesies have not rallied the faithful. None of these theories have compelled large numbers of sleep researchers to say "I believe. Yes, this is the function of sleep." We wait for more evidence. What kind of evidence? What do we want? That is what this paper is about --the kind of evidence we will require to convince each other about the function of sleep. Our discussion might well begin with a brief review of what we mean by need or function and of how we deal with it scientifically.

THE CONCEPT OF NEED

Although needs or functions may be defined by empirical measures, these measures are usually guided by concepts of need. In our effort to estimate truths beyond what is empirically known, we are forever generating concepts (i.e., ideas, hypotheses, theories) which organize and elaborate upon old facts and hopefully guide us to new facts. Our ordinary concept of function in biology is that life processes or interactions with the environment periodically create states or needs which threaten the organism's welfare. These needs act as stimuli for corrective mechanisms which generate activities or consummatory responses that alleviate the need.

The success of a concept is evaluated by the number of different facts which it encompasses-- both old facts and new facts which emerge from research generated by the concept. The concept of need has been very successful in some areas. It has, for example, been able to connect facts about stimulus conditions (e.g., giving or withholding of food), organic deficit (e.g., cell damage and weight loss), behavioral deficit (e.g., motor weakness), sensing mechanisms (e.g., satiey centers), consummatory activity (e.g., eating and digestion), and reversal of deficits after compensatory consummation.

Several features of sleep suggest but cannot guarantee in advance, that it could be successfully conceptualized as a consummatory activity:

the ubiquitousness of sleep across species and
within individuals; the periodic occurrence of
sleep; the effects of sleep deprivation; the reversal of deficits after recovery of sleep; the
correlations between sleep and fundamental biological parameters (Zepelin & Rechtschaffen, 1974).
To know the function of sleep would mean to identify with confidence the specific state of maladaptiveness or need which sleep alleviates. A
more complete understanding of the functional
system as a whole would include knowledge of how
this maladaptiveness stimulates sleep mechanisms,
how these mechanisms produce sleep, and what it is
about sleep that alleviates the condition of need.
The relationship between the search for function
and the search for mechanism cannot be decided
a priori. Conceivably, considerable understanding
of either could be achieved independent of the
other. One could understand why sleep is adaptive
without understanding how it is produced, and
vice versa. More likely, the two searches would
be mutually enhancing. Clues to mechanisms can
come from knowing the need conditions which should
stimulate the mechanisms and the "directions" in
which the mechanisms had to move to satisfy need.
Clues to function could come from knowing how
mechanisms were activated and the apparent
"directions" in which they were moving. Some may
wonder whether there is merit in invoking the
concept of need at all, whether the whole issue
could not be approached less teleologically in
terms of mechanism alone. Our preferred response
is that function is simply a convenient, short-
hand way of referring to the data of survival and
propagation, the conditions which favor and reduce
them, and the mechanisms of natural selection
which determine the responses to these conditions.
Need really refers to a class of data and
mechanisms, with no mysterious notions of purpose
intended.
   The success of a concept depends upon its
interaction with empirical observations. Empirical
information shapes the formation of concepts which
in turn may guide the selection of empirical information. For example, the concept of need for
food was generated in antiquity by commonplace
observations of relationships among lack of food,
consequent deficits, subjective desires,

compensatory consummation, and reversal of deficits
after consummation. These relationships were
sufficiently strong that one could then use any one
of a number of empirical measures to designate the
need" amount of food eaten; reports of desire for
food; weight loss, etc. Each of these manifestly
different observables could be used as a measure of
the theoretical concept of need for food. Almost
inevitably, however, empirical observations arise
which do violence to the concept; they do not fit
into the network of relationships from which need
was inferred. For example, there may be no organ
deficits following prolonged food deprivation, as
in the case of prior obesity, or deficits may occur
in spite of abundant eating, as when one eats the
"wrong foods". At this point one may change the
concept because it does not fit the empirical observations, or one may reject the discordant observations under the rationale that in some situations
empirical data may yield poor estimations of the
concept. The best outcomes are when concepts or
measures or both can be changed to become more
concordant, e.g., as when the need for food becomes
identified more specifically as a need for certain
nutritional substances. Under this revised concept,
food intake per se becomes only a very crude and
sometimes misleading indicator of the revised
concept of need for nutritional substances.

The important point for us now is that the
choice of empirical referents for the sleep need
can sometimes be very misleading, not only with
respect to what that need may eventually turn out
to be, but also in the initial recognition of when
a state of need exists. In some cases the choice
of empirical referent may do violence to the very
concept of need itself. We will try to illustrate
these problems more specifically later, but first
we may take note of the problems which arise from
the limitations of empirical data.

EMPIRICAL INFORMATION

Fundamentally, the scientist gathers three
kinds of empirical information; each has its
intrinsic limitations. 1. Description. This
includes the selection of target phenomena, development of the methods of reliable measurement, and
organization of the observations for public presentation. The choice of phenomena to be described
as indicative of need for sleep is largely a matter

conceptual strategy, inference, guess, and luck.
Once having chosen a selected phenomenon for description, the task remains of relating it to other
variables. It is here that we run into methodological limitations over and above the problem of
concept formation and definition. 2. Response
correlation. Here the researcher determines the
relationship between responses, including those
which occur spontaneously and those which occur in
response to standard stimuli. Relatively static
variables such as organism structure may be
considered as responses to prior genetic, growth
and adaptational history. Response correlation, at
least in the case of spontaneous responses, has the
merit of dealing with naturally occurring activity,
the activity we usually want to explain, but it
tells us little about causality. A correlation
between two responses leaves unresolved the question of which variable is affecting the other, or
whether the two are related by virtue of a third
variable which is causal to both of them. 3.
Stimulus manipulation. Here the researcher determines the effect of his active manipulation of
stimulus conditions on responses. This strategy
permits conclusions about cause and effect--but
only about the effect of the stimuli upon responses.
A frequent overinterpretation is the claim that one
response to the stimulus causes or mediates a final
response of interest. Stimuli produce several internal responses; which of these causally mediate a
final response of interest is a matter of interpretation. It is crucial that the stimuli be experimentally modified for causality to be established;
naturally occurring variations are responses to
other, frequently unknown, variables which could be
the causal determinants. Another limitation of the
stimulus-response strategy is that the responses to
the stimuli may not be the same as the naturally
occurring responses of interest.

Now we may consider how these limitations of
empirical data together with the problems of conceptualization bear more specifically on the different strategies used to search for sleep function.
Much recent research has focused on the functions
of specific sleep stages. Since our discussion is
about research strategies rather than specific
results, we need not complicate the discussion un-
necessarily by considering individual stages. For

the most part, the research principles discussed
here would apply equally well to the search for
specific sleep stage functions.

SLEEP DEPRIVATION

One obvious strategy for getting at the
function of sleep is to see what goes wrong when
we do not have it, i.e., sleep deprivation experi-
ments.First we encounter a methodological limitation. In the sleep deprivation paradigm, we cannot
conclusively establish the effects of sleep deprivation; rather, we establish the correlates of sleep
deprivation, from which one may or may not hypothesize causal effects. The sleep deprivation
study is a stimulus manipulation experiment in which
the experimenter does something, such as keep a
rat on a water wheel, to maintain wakefulness. The
procedure used to keep the animal awake, not the
wakefulness per se is the experimentally manipu-
lated stimulus and therefore the only certain
causal agent. This causal agent produces two
responses. One response is prolonged wakefulness.
The other response, in many instances, is a functional or structural deficit. It is easy to slip
into the assumption that one of the responses,
sleep deprivation, was causal to the other, the
deficit. This may or may not be true, but it is
not proven. Both responses might be produced by
the stimulus without either response affecting the
other. Several days on a water wheel could produce
both wakefulness and several chemical, behavioral,
or structural deficits. The deficits could result
either from the sleep deprivation or from the
stress of the water wheel independent of sleep loss.
Which deficits result from sleep loss and which
deficits result from the procedures used to induce
sleep loss cannot be clearly separated by sleep
deprivation experiments alone. In human studies,
Taub and Berger (1973) have shown that relatively
small manipulations of circadian rhythm can be much
more disruptive to mood and performance than small
amounts of sleep deprivation. Since sleep deprivation studies always involve a disruption of rhythm,
it is risky to attribute the resulting deficits to
loss of sleep per se.
     A second problem with the sleep deprivation
experiment is a conceptual one--the interpretation

of the presumed deficit. An assault on organisms'
adaptiveness may be followed not only by functional
deficit, but very often by homeostatic, compensatory
reactions which militate for restored adaptation
or maximization of overall effectiveness under
conditions of impairment. Sometimes it is difficult
to distinguish an impairment from an adaptive
response to the impairment. For example, a frequent
correlate of sleep deprivation in humans is impaired
performance on intellectual and psychomotor tasks
which frequently takes the form of lapses of attention. Such data naturally invite the interpretation that sleep is important for restoring the
brain's capacity to process data, store information,
etc. However, the lapses in performance efficiency
could result from incipient sleep processes which
are adaptive responses to insufficient sleep. This
does not deny that there is a performance deficit,
but the deficit may reveal more about adaptation
to sleep loss than about the function of sleep. To
accept the adaptive response as the indicator of
sleep function is tantamount to saying that the
function of sleep is to keep us from being sleepy.
This answer misses the point of searching for
function, i.e., to relate an activity, by virtue of
its adaptiveness, to variables other than itself.

The issue of sleepiness raises a conceptual
problem about the effectiveness of the deprivation
procedure. There are two ways of conceptualizing
the sleepiness which almost inevitably occurs
during sleep deprivation procedures. One is to see
sleepiness as sleep preparatory behavior we have to
go through before realizing the benefit of sleep
itself--just as we have to obtain and swallow our
food before we can enjoy nutritional benefits. In
this conceptualization, the deprivation procedures
permit the preparatory responses while preventing
the consummatory response of sleep itself. Another
view is to see sleepiness as partial sleep. After
all, the two states do have much in common--
decreased vigilance, motor relaxation, eye closure,
etc. Under this view, sleepiness is a mini-
consummatory event. It is more analogous to having
a snack than it is to cooking. If this view is
correct, it could mean that the experimental procedures which aim to prevent sleep are not very
effective. This alternative may not be very
serious for sleep deprivation experiments which

produce deficits in addition to sleepiness per se,
but it is a problem for experiments that yield no
substantial consequences apart from sleepiness.
Unfortunately, the problem is more often the case.
Think of how easy it is to experimentally induce
sleepiness but how difficult it has been to show
other consequences of sleep deprivation. It could
be counter-argued that the fact of induced
sleepiness demonstrates the effectiveness of the
deprivation procedure. On the other hand, we know
that in other need systems, e.g., food, that consummation may be stimulated by deprivation which
is too mild to produce damage of any consequence.
In fact, it should be the earmark of any successful need system to produce adaptive reactions long
before any damage is done.

These considerations challenge our ingenuity,
i.e., how to produce a sleep deprived state by
procedures which are gentle enough not to seriously
disrupt the subject in other ways but which are
potent enough to prevent partial sleep.

To summarize, sleep deprivation experiments
leave us with several ambiguities. First we may
wonder how well they prevented sleep. Second,
assuming sleep was adequately reduced, were the
deficits really deficits? Third, even assuming
they are deficits, were they produced by the sleep
deprivation?

STIMULATION EXPERIMENTS

When we use stimulus manipulation to get at
function, most often we implicitly or explicitly
infer that the stimulus manipulation changed the
internal need for sleep--either increasing it to
increase sleep or decreasing it to decrease sleep.
Although we may be sure that the external stimulus
manipulations were causal, we cannot be sure about
which mediating responses produced by the stimuli
affected the final response. The problem arises
when the zealous theorist does not recognize alternative interpretations, beside need state, which
could explain the effect of the stimuli. One
alternative is that the mechanisms for sleep or
wakefulness may be directly stimulated while by-
passing the internal need states which normally
produce these responses, as when food intake is

stimulated in the absence of any real need for food.
Rhythmic sounds can be soporific. Does that mean
that the function of sleep is to cope with rhythmic
stimulation? No, we fall asleep every night no
matter what the beat. Possibly, rhythm directly
stimulates sleep mechanisms independent of need.
We know that sleep sated animals can be made to
sleep with appropriate drugs, presumably through
their direct action on the mechanisms of sleep or
wakefulness. Why should not similar effects be
possible with external stimuli?

The direct effect of stimulus manipulation can
reach its most drastic form when the mechanisms is
rendered virtually inoperative. For example, if
animals sleep less in extreme heat or extreme cold,
it does not necessarily mean that the function of
sleep is to help maintain a certain body or brain
temperature and that sleep was reduced because the
need was met by the experimental manipulation of
temperature. Rather, it could mean that sleep
mechanisms, like so many others, work best under
relatively narrow conditions of the internal and
external environment.

As noted earlier, responses to experimental
stimuli may not be equivalent to the naturally
occurring responses we wish to explain. This has
not been a major problem in the manipulation of
sleep by the external environment, simply because
such manipulations generally have not had very
great or consistent effects on sleep. Also, if
the manipulations are within the limits of ordinary
environmental circumstances, it is unlikely that
the sleep they produced would be extraordinary.
The problem is greater when surgical, chemical, or
electrical stimulation of the brain has been used.
To use the results of such drastic interventions
as evidence on the function of sleep can be risky.
The non-physiologic character of these interventions,
such as the administration of electrical impulses
several times more intense than any electrical
activity which occurs normally in the brain, should
in itself give rise to skepticism about whether the
sleep or wakefulness that is induced is normal.
In addition, there is more direct evidence of response artificiality. Some of the brain lesions
which reduced sleep also cause the redistribution
of ponto-geniculate-occipital spikes within sleep
and their appearance in large numbers during

wakefulness. Lesions which induce apparent sleep
are always suspect as having produced states of
debilitation, unresponsiveness, or coma which may
be very different from normal sleep. The differences between drug induced and natural sleep or
wakefulness have been discussed too often to
warrant further comment here.

RESPONSE CORRELATION

The pitfalls of inferences about sleep function
from response correlations are usually too obvious
to warrant more than brief comment. In each case,
the correlation between two variables leaves un-
answered the question of which variable, if either,
was causal, or whether a third variable was causal
to both.

One obvious response correlation strategy is
to observe which other responses are simultaneous
with or absent during the sleep response. The
implicit or explicit rationale is that sleep is in
the service of the other response or lack of it.
For example, physical rest is a very obvious correlate of sleep, which is no doubt responsible for
the widespread idea that the function of sleep is
rest. However, it is clear that physical rest may
occur independent of sleep without the price of
loss of vigilance that sleep entails, that a night
of rest without sleep does not substitute for sleep,
and that sleep does not vary very much in the face
of huge day to day variations in physical activity.
The physical rest which regularly accompanies sleep
may be in the service of sleep rather than the
other way around. Rest may facilitate or permit the
operation of the mechanisms of sleep which fill a
function quite unrelated to rest. In other words,
we may rest to sleep rather than sleep to rest. The
possibility is not far-fetched. For example, the
purpose of elimination is not to rest our legs, although the two responses are almost perfectly correlated.

Many scientists who are too sophisticated to
infer causality from correlated simultaneous responses will slip into cause-effect conclusions if
one of the responses regularly precedes the other.
For example, the fact that feelings of fatigue frequently precede sleep can lead to the interpretation that we sleep because we are fatigued.

However, the fact that one response precedes another
is no guarantee that the first is causal to the
second. A third variable may independently initiate
both responses, but the processes leading to one
may take longer than the processes leading to the
other. Also, the first response may simply be an
early manifestation of the second. The fatigue we
feel before sleep may simply be the first overt
signs that the sleep process has begun. What we
experience as pre-sleep fatigue may be incipient
sleepiness--not a cause of sleep.

A parallel problem obtains for responses which
follow sleep. In this case, the implicit or explicit reasoning is that the function of sleep is
revealed by how we have changed after sleep. For
example, the quantity and quality of sleep may be
correlated with the elevation of mood the following morning. Such correlations could suggest that
the function of sleep is to somehow attenuate or
resolve problems that remain in the psyche at the
end of the day. However, some dissipation of problems prior to sleep could have caused both the
good night of sleep and the morning elevation of
mood. Also, intellectual performance may improve
following sleep because sleep preparatory responses
no longer compete with task oriented responses, not
because the function of sleep necessarily has anything to do with intellectual work.

Much of the research on relationships between
sleep and subject differences, including species,
age, intelligence, personality, etc., has suggested theories of the function of sleep or of specific
sleep stages. The most frequent kind of hypothesis
is that individuals who sleep the most do so because
they need it most. The apparent working assumption
is that the need is being satisfied. Most theorists
have recognized the correlative nature of the
data, but sometimes with only passing lip service
to alternative interpretations which may be very
reasonable. Some subjects or groups might sleep
much not because they need it most but because
they have the best developed or functioning
mechanisms for getting it. They may be the
subjects who need sleep the least. Anomalies
in long sleepers could be the result of too much
sleep--not too little sleep, i.e., sleep might be
the cause, not the effect of other subject characteristics. Also, both the sleep and the other subject

characteristics could be correlated but separately caused results of unknown genetic, developmental, or historical variables.

SLEEP SUBSTITUTION

A potentially powerful strategy for understanding the need for sleep is to find stimulus conditions or responses which appear to do away with it. Operationally this means discovering something we can do to or for the subject or something he does for himself which enables him to get along very well without it or with very little of it--figuratively speaking, intravenous sleep. This strategy involves conceptual and methodological questions similar to those raised earlier. Did the putative substitute really stop sleep? Was the need fulfilled or was the mechanism blocked? One new question emerges. Is sleep necessary? It has been reported that some individuals or species sleep very little or even not at all, yet appear to live reasonably healthy, normal lives (see Meddis, 1975 for review). This information invites two different perspectives. One suggests that the concept that sleep filled some need has been over-emphasized, that sleep may not fill a need. This perspective implies the burden of finding a new concept that organizes as many facts about sleep as the need concept does, including the phenomenon of rebound after sleep deprivation. The second perspective suggests that the need which was ordinarily fulfilled by sleep was being fulfilled in short sleeping individuals or groups by mechanisms which did not produce the full blown behaviors or electrographic characteristics of sleep. These individuals would then be seen as the proverbial "experiments in nature" and could occasion intense investigations in a search for sleep substitutes. Such studies could help us resolve which aspects of sleep were need fulfilling and which were epi-phenomenal to need fulfillment.

INTEGRATION

To this point our discussion appears a bit nihilistic. Every individual bit of evidence on the function of sleep seems vulnerable to alternative interpretations--either because of the uncertain relationship between the concept of function and its empirical referents or because of the intrinsic limitations of research methods. Is there any hope? Yes, the answer is in a multiplicity of empirical measures and research strategies. Fortunately, the sins of one measure are not necessarily visited upon the next. As the network of relationships among different measures and results from different strategies expands in number and variety, those emerging interpretations which fit the network best become favored over alternative interpretations which are measure or method specific.

To illustrate, we can hypothesize that sleep is necessary as the neural state most compatible with the synthesis of chemical X, which is catabolized at high rates during wakefulness in the service of other functions. Suppose we then accumulated the following results: Sleep deprivation produces a deficiency of X and, after a period of delay, physiological symptoms. Administration of X after deprivation eliminates the sleepiness, the sleep rebound, and the physiological symptoms which normally follow sleep deprivation. Drugs which augment synthesis of X reduce sleep without signs of the physiological symptoms of sleep deprivation. Drugs which block the synthesis of X increase sleep. Drugs which block catabolism of X decrease sleep but produce the physiological symptoms of sleep deprivation. Stimulus conditions which increase the catabolism of X produce an increase in sleep. Species, age groups, and individuals which catabolize X the fastest sleep the most. Individuals who do not sleep synthesize X at high rates during wakefulness.

If all of this came to pass, then we would believe that the function of sleep was the synthesis of X. Each individual result would still be open to alternative interpretations. One could still wonder in the sleep deprivation experiments whether the reduction of X was attributable to the loss of sleep or more directly to the procedures used to prevent sleep and whether the physiological symptoms were attributable to the reduction of X or to some other consequence of the procedure. In the pharmacological studies one could still wonder whether the effects of the various drugs on sleep and

symptoms were truly mediated by their effects on X
or by other actions such as direct control of sleep
mechanisms. In the correlational studies one could
still wonder whether individual characteristics
were the cause or the effect of their correlations
with sleep and X, or whether a third variable was
causal to all three. In any individual study one
could still question the appropriateness of any
single empirical referent of sleep need, total
sleep, or functional deficit. However, a rejection
of the X-theory of sleep function, given the network of relationships described above, would be
tantamount to choosing a different anti-X interpretation in each of the individual studies. In
some cases we would be rejecting X-theory because
we favored the interpretation that stimuli which
affected X and sleep were acting independently on
the two responses. In other cases we would be
rejecting X-theory because we favored the interpretation that correlations between X and sleep did
not reflect causal relationships between them. In
still other cases we would be rejecting X-theory
because we did not think that sleep or functional
deficit were adequately defined by the empirical
measures. A rejection of X-theory would then
constitute an unparsimonious array of different
interpretations compared to the neat parsimony of
X-theory. Under these circumstances we would
rather accept X-theory until an even more parsimonious idea came along--and that is as close as
we can come to believing any theory which includes
non-empirical terms.

The example of X-theory should not be taken
as a bias for chemical restoration theories of
sleep. This model was chosen simply because it
was easy to discuss, and people are accustomed to
thinking about chemical restoration. The advan-
tages of multiple lines of converging evidence
would apply in the case of other kinds of theories
as well, including conservation and behaviorally
oriented theories. Of course, some theories may
suffer limitations in the availability of varieties
of evidence. For example, for those theories in
which sleep is a response to the natural selection
history of the species but not necessarily to
immediate environmental or biological circumstances
of individuals, relevant stimulus manipulation

experiments would be most difficult (e.g., comparing genetic histories under different imposed
environments, or comparing survival rates under
various circumstances in animals selectively bred
for high and low sleep quotas.)

Now we may return to our original question
about the kind of evidence we want before we accept
a theory of sleep function. We want converging
evidence from a number of different empirical
measures because each individual measure can be
variously interpreted as to what it signifies about
need, deficit, or sleep. We also want evidence from
a number of different research strategies because
the results from any single strategy can be variously interpreted in terms of causal relationships.

This perspective suggests that theories of sleep
function should be offered rather modestly until
they are supported by evidence from several research
strategies. This consideration is a double-edged
sword. On the one hand we have skeptical reserve
about the significance of any individual fact. On
the other hand the acceptable theory must come from
the collection of individual facts. Thus it would
be a mistake for a granting agency to reject a research proposal on the function of sleep because
the result would not decisively resolve the issue
of sleep function. No single result will resolve
the issue, and any individual result, negative or
positive, can be important information for the
theoretical network. For the researcher, a recognition of the inevitable ambiguity of single experiments should dampen interminable arguments about
their decisiveness. With luck, an individual experiment might uncover the function of sleep, but it
could not prove it. On the other hand, a recognition of the value of single experiments can esca-
late into the old defense of heurism as the basis
for suggesting theories from individual experiments.
It is a valid argument in principle, but a judgment
call in individual cases. It is a question of how
big a deal one makes out of how little information.
There is a dividing line over which one can pass
from heurism to baloney.

A second implication is that, since an acceptable theory of sleep function will depend upon a
network of information, it is crucial that the
theoretician consider all the evidence relevant to
the theory--both positive and negative. The outright neglect of negative evidence is, I believe,

relatively rare and easily detected. More ominous
is the failure to give equal attention to negative
results and the dismissal of negative results as
special idiosyncratic cases without a concomitant
constriction of the generality of the theory. An
especially dastardly tactic, because it converts
evidence against a theory into evidence apparently
supportive of it, is the citation of research reports as being "in the right direction", whereas
inspection of the original data reveals only a non-
significant, miniscule edge leaning towards the
theory's side. If all of this sounds a bit moral-
istic, be assured that our thrust is not so much
against sin--which can be a lot of fun--but against
dilution of the joy in our search by distracting
cheap shots. We started this paper by noting our
good fortune in having such an important question
as the function of sleep. If it is a glorious
question, it deserves a glorious answer, not an
inflation of limited data to cosmic generalizations
or the biased review of relevant data.

     We have deliberately avoided a substantive
review of any specific theory of sleep function.
We think that some have been lightweight and others
have been sincere contributions--whether we agree
with them or not. We leave it to the readers to
decide for themselves. There was not enough time
for us to do equal injustice to them all.

     Finally, we would like to express our mis-
givings about papers such as this. We would rather
have presented a theory of our own we thought was
worth presenting, but we do not have one. Methodological analyses like this help us understand our
ignorance, but they rarely increase our knowledge.
This analysis is not a guide to the solution of
the function of sleep; it is more a scencario of
how diverse information will fall into place when
the answer comes. The answer will not come from
checking lists of possible misinterpretations, but
from a new idea or result which suddenly coalesces
our facts and fancies. It will probably come at
four in the morning in a dingy laboratory in
Minneapolis to a graduate student in biology who
never read this paper. God bless him.

ACKNOWLEDGMENT

Supported by National Institute of Mental Health Grants M-4151 and MH-K3-18428

REFERENCES

Meddis, R. On the function of sleep. Animal Behavior, 23, 676-691, 1975.

Taub, J. M. and Berger, R. J. Performance and mood following variations in the length and timing of sleep. Psychophysiology, 10, 559-570, 1973.

Zepelin, H. and Rechtschaffen, A. Mammalian sleep, longevity, and energy metabolism. Brain, Behavior and Evolution, 10, 425-470, 1974.

THEORIES OF SLEEP FUNCTIONS AND SOME CLINICAL IMPLICATIONS

WILSE B. WEBB

Department of Psychology
University of Florida
Gainesville, Florida

According to the French philosopher, physicist and historian, Pierre Duhem (1954), Plato in his Republic argued that there were three kinds of truths - observational, geometrical and philosophical. The first is given by our sense perceptions, the second our reasoning, and the third by "pure intellect." Relative to sleep research the first is referent to our descriptive observations - stages do exist, biochemical changes are present, animals sleep differently. The second level refers to our finding systematic interrelationships and organizing them into rubrics --- REM rebounds under deprivation, Stage 4 diminishes with age, sleep varies relative to serotonin levels --- "the erratic patterns of the stars seen by the eye take on simple and consistent orbits. The third level is concerned with "why" or "to what ends".

The facts about sleep have burgeoned in the past two decades in the modern era of Sleep Research which began in the late 1950's (Webb, 1973; Williams, et al, 1973). In 1968 this research was described as "almost exclusively a-theoretical in its general approach and diligently devoted to the collection of empirical facts" (Webb, 1968, p. 56). While the accepting caveat that "theorizing without basic data is (a) futile enterprise," concern was expressed about our failure to approach the problems propounded by Samuel Johnson more than 300 years ago: "No searcher has yet found either the efficient or final cause...or what benefits the animal receives from this alternate suspension of its active powers."

Recently several distinct positions have emerged about the function of sleep or, more specifically, why sleep is present in the behavior of animals. This paper will review these theories.[1]

A search for the purposes of sleep is complicated by the problem of levels of explanation which

Copyright © 1979 by Academic Press, Inc.
All rights of reproduction in any form reserved.
ISBN 0-12-222340-3

is echoed in Johnson's early quoted statements;
"efficient or final cause." There have been a
plethora of statements about "efficient" or
"partial" causes of sleep (Snyder, 1962). These
extend, at least, from Aristotle's attribution of
sleep to the cooling of vapor in the head
(Aristotle, 1951) through the presence of "toxins"
(Kleitman, 1963) to current findings relative to
biochemical changes in the central nervous system
(Jouvet, 1967). Most of these efforts have been
focussed on an "efficient" cause of sleep, i.e.,
the immediate antecedents to the onset of sleep.
There has been, in addition, the development of a
different form of "partial" theories to account for
the specific role of that segment of sleep variously
designated as "REM" (rapid eye movement), "paradoxical" or "activated" sleep. Considerable experimental work and theorizing has been focussed on
the function of this phase of sleep (Fishbein &
Gutwein, 1977; Greenberg & Pearlman, 1974).

Certainly the "efficient" causes of sleep in
terms of immediate or concurrent mechanisms are
relevant to sleep presence. The functional effect
of REM sleep within sleep may be an "efficient"
role of sleep (and some argue as the necessary
cause of sleep). However, in this review we focus
on higher order theories concerned with "final"
causes-why the animal sleeps. Or again, invoking
Johnson: "...what benefits the animal receives
from this alternate suspension of its active
powers."

At least five general positions of some contemporary force can be recognized. While presented
as distinct and independent positions for expository
purposes we will see that they are often mixed in
various combinations. An attempt has been made to
present each theory positively with its primary
data base.

                    THE RESTORATIVE THEORY

This position holds that sleep is a period of
recovery or restoration of physiological, neurological and/or psychological states. The position
implicitly underlies the earlier "toxin" theories
of sleep and is certainly the widely held intuitive
notion about sleep. As Hartmann puts it, "...to
the layman, Why do we sleep? is a natural question,

and he even has an answer though in very vague
terms: sleep restores" (Hartman, 1973, p. 3).
    Hartmann (1973), Oswald (1970, 1974) and
Moruzzi (1966, 1972) have most completely articulated the restorative positions. Oswald
summarizes the position by a quotation from
Shakespeare's Macbeth: "Sore labour's bath, balm
of hurt minds...chief nourisher in life's feast..."
Both Hartmann and Oswald view nonREM or slow wave
sleep (SWS) as restorative of "physical" of
"general bodily tissues" and ascribe to REM sleep
"cortical" or "brain" restorative functions.
Moruzzi, on the other hand, denigrates the
restorarive properties of sleep relative to the
skeletal muscles, visceral organs or the autonomic
nervous system but details the restorative functions
associated with "not the whole cerebrum, nor even
the entire neocortex, but only those neurons or
synapses, and possible glia cells, which during
wakefulness are responsible for, or are related
to, the brain functions concerned conscious
behavior" (1972, p. 121). More specifically
Moruzzi refers to those synapses associated with
learning and memory.
    Certainly the most powerful supportive founda-
tion stone of the restorative theories is that
titled by Hartmann "The Psychology of Tiredness"
-we feel tired before we go to sleep and rested or
recovered after sleep. The experimental support
for this position of physical recovery relates to
the conditions which allegedly are associated with
the increase in SWS and human growth hormone: prolonged wakefulness, exercise, fasting, hyperthyro-
dism and the association of high and low SWS
amounts with developmental changes of growth and
aging (Hartmann, 1973; Oswald, 1974). The biochemical supportive arguments center on the increased rates of mitosis and protein synthesis
rates associated with rest and sleep (Adams &
Oswald, 1976). Moruzzi presents an elaborate
neurophysiological schema which relates the
presence of cortical inhibitory processes, particularly during the desynchronized (REM) phases of
sleep with the potential for slow recovery processes for those synapses "where plastic (macro-
molecular) changes occur during wakefulness, as a
consequence of higher nervous activities such as

those involved in learning or conditioning"
(Moruzzi, 1966, p.376).

THE PROTECTIVE THEORIES

This position asserts that the function of sleep
is to protect the organism from excessive wear and
tear. As early stated by Claparede, "We do not
sleep because we are exhausted but to avoid becoming exhausted" (1905). Pavlov, in response to
the continuous elicitation of sleep in his classical conditioning experiments, developed his
protective theory: "...The progressively developing inhibition, which itself can be regarded as
a functional extinction, but which is the result
of exhaustion, assumes the role of a protector of
cortical elements, preventing any excessive fatigue
or dangerous functional destruction... Such a
state of widely spread inhibition actually does
occur exactly in the same manner as in the case of
the individual cortical elements, and is familiar
to all of us as the common and everyday occurrence
of sleep... Sleep and what we call internal inhibition are one and the same process" (Pavlov, 1927,
p. 250). From his experimental data he concluded
that sleep then was a diffusion of cortical inhibition over the cortex which served to protect the
cortical system from exhaustion.

Pavlov's notions as well as the earlier de-
activation theories of sleep were confounded by
the detailed analyses of the neurophysiology of
sleep initiated by the work of Moruzzi and Magoun
(1949). These intensive investigations were
summarized by Moruzzi in 1966 (p. 346):

"Summing up, even during the less active phase
of sleep the neurons of the motor and visual
cortices never rest; indeed, some of them seem to
be paradoxically, more active during synchronized
sleep than during relaxed wakefulness. A further
phasic enhancement of their activity occurs during
the desynchronized phase".

Moruzzi, as noted above, however, does espouse
a form of inhibitory hypothesis of sleep:

"...the mass inhibition of cortical neurons
which Pavlov had postulated certainly does not
exist, but it would be impossible to deny that
some neurons of the ascending reticular system
share the same properties of the interneurons of

the cerebrum with regard to the need for prolonged periods of rest" (1962, p. 378).

THE ENERGY CONSERVATION HYPOTHESIS

This position holds that the function of sleep is to conserve energy. This is a corollary of the reported correlation of estimated total sleep time and metabolic rate of .65 in 29 species of animals (Zepelin & Rechtshaffen, 1974). As the authors state: "The correlation between sleep time and metabolic rate suggests that sleep has the function of enforcing rest and limiting metabolic requirements..."

These data are supportive of two earlier statements regarding sleep and metabolism which were derived from evolutionary considerations. The phylogenetic data provided indications that while all mammals and birds present evidence of SWS as measured by EEG, amphibians such as bull, frogs and salamanders did not and the presence of EEG indexed sleep in reptiles such as lizards, chameleons, and turtles was not present or equivocal. From these observations and evolutionary history it was concluded that: "...The descendants of reptiles-the mammals and the birds-have two things in common: they both sleep, and they both maintain constant body temperatures despite changes in environmental temperature. The ability of the mammals and birds to be active at any temperature is a distinct advantage over reptiles.. A disadvantage in this mechanism, though, is that a great deal of food is required to keep the mammal or bird body warm; it would be advantageous to turn down their body thermostat when the stomach is full or danger is not imminent... Slow wave sleep may have evolved parallel with temperature regulation, as an active brain mechanism in the brain or periodically "forcing" mammals and birds-with their generally high body temperature-to conserve energy" (Allison & Van Twyver, 1970, p. 60).

Berger, also reviewing phylogenetic data, similarly concludes that "sleep constitutes a period of dormancy in which energy is conserved to partially offset the increased energy demands of homeostasis" (Berger, 1975).

THE ETHOLOGICAL THEORY

Two essentially parallel statements of this theory have been made by Meddis (1975, 1977) and by Webb (1971, 1974a, 1974b, 1975) A similar set of conceptualizations was expressed by Snyder (1972). The position holds that the role of sleep is a control system of behavior to enhance survical. This position may also be labelled "adaptive."

There are two primary postulates. First, there are environmental pressures, differing in the ecology of each species, that make nonresponding a salient factor in survival and, secondly, sleep serves as a necessary state to aid and maintain these periods of non-responding. This theory draws its data from phylogenetic sleep patterns which display a range total sleep from possibly no sleep (Dall Porpoise) through certainly limited sleep amounts of between 2 to 4 hours displayed by horses and such grazing animals as cattle, goats, elephants and sheep to large amounts of sleep of more than 15 hours found in such species as opposums and sloths; highly intermittant to long sleep periods and variations in the placement of sleep within the twenty-four hours. From these variations, the ethological position argues that each sleep pattern evolved as adaptive systems which enhanced survival by increasing the safety and energy gathering (foraging) behavior of each species relative to their ecological niche.

Sleep on one hand removes the animal from ecologically maladaptive periods of time and on the other hand non sleep permits maintenance of effective survival activities. These theories take from Shakespeare's Hamlet their theme: "What is man if his chief good and market be but to sleep and feed?"

THE INSTINCTIVE THEORY

This position considers sleep to be an instinct, i.e., a species specific, innate, organized pattern of behavior which is elicited in the presence of particular cues. The function of sleep then, like migration, nest building or imprinting, is considered to be an expression or fulfillment of behavior rather than a "need" recovery or "drive" reduction behavior.

The most extensive treatment of this concept is given by Moruzzi (1966, 1972). He finds it necessary to reject a simple homeostatic need-need reduction concept, e.g., regulated maintenance of a fixed internal environment such as a constancy of "water and salt contents or O_2 and CO_2 tensions. He notes that the presence of feedback controls in sleep are much looser than is typical of the classical homeostatic systems and finds little likelihood of "feedback regulation from structures which benefit of the sleep recovery." As a consequence he postulates that the protective-restorative homeostasis (which he further hypothesizes) is maintained by functionally integrated patterns of instinctive behavior. These in turn are the result of "more or less stereotyped spatio-temporal patterns of moto-neuron discharge" which elicits functionally appropriate sleep behavior.

McGinty, reasoning from neurophysiological data, stated a similar set of proposals in 1971 (McGinty, 1971). He summarized these recently (McGinty et al, 1974, p. 181): "...We believe that neural control of SWS in mammals is most satisfactorily conceived by comparison with complex appetitive behavior such as feeding, and courtship ...complex instinctive behavior or reflexive components such as the lordosis reflex, sham rage, or REM sleep, are organized at the level of the brain stem ...Diencephalic structures have been implicated in cyclic patterns of behavior (and) quantitive regulation regulation of consumption ...limbic and neocortical systems control the selective of appropriate goals objects...voluntary motor behaviors which prepare the organism for "consumption,"...learned adaptation to the environment and perceptual controls over behavior..."

The clear interrelationship between this position and the ethological theories is seen in the discussion of these theories in which the instinctive model is made a part of the more general ethological theories (McGinty, 1974; Webb, 1974b). Indeed, Moruzzi, in consideration of the wide range of sleep behavior patterns across species, concludes that there are "...some serious reasons to believe that the instinctive component is of paramount importance and that the sleep-waking cycle is dominated by it, rather than by

the neurochemical requirements of the brain... The
needs of brain recovery do not represent the only,
or probably even a major factor, in the regulation
of the sleep-wake cycle" (Moruzzi, 1972, pp. 133-
134).

INTERTWINNINGS

The five positions outlined have been presented
in independent groupings. But certainly in the
presentations the combinations of positions could
be seen as possible and, in certain writers,
present. The relationships, in fact, range from
statements of outright opposition through varying
combinations.

The ethological theories of sleep have tended
to be stated as alternatives to the restorative
theories of sleep. Perhaps part of this stems from
the sometimes explicit statements that sleep is a
non-adaptive state and hence important restorative
activities must be present to justify this
"dangerous" condition. This was explicitly stated
by a doyen of the recuperative theorists, Hess:

"During sleep these capacities (reactivity to
signals) are depressed and the individual is left
helpless... (to) accept this risk for a considerable part of their life suggests that sleep must
be a vital function. We consider it a reparative
process" (Hess, 1954, p. 117).

Meddis from his ethological position flatly
states: "...such theories must explain, firstly,
what this process of restitution is, and secondly,
why it is required in large quantities by some
species and hardly at all by others... the burden
of proof must remain with the recuperation theories"
(Meddis, 1975, p. 684). Webb, while admitting
the possibilities of "restoration," finds such
arguments orthogonal to his adaptive approach but
complains of the "non predictive" quality of restoration theories (Webb, 1974b).

Even within given positions there are dis-
agreements. Within the restorative theories both
Hartmann and Oswald specify a "bodily" recovery
process while Moruzzi states: "It is easy to show
that the aim of sleep is not to give a period of
rest to skeletal muscles of visceral organs, not
to permit the recovery of the spinal cord and of
the autonomic nervous system...most hypnic

symptoms are in fact epiphenomena: Their
importance is magnified by our unconscious anthropomorphic attitude: (Moruzzi, 1972, p. 121).
    But monolithic positions are less common than
one or more being offered in combination. Moruzzi,
in fact, can be said to combine all the positions
as he suggests that sleep 1) begins with drowsiness
which elicits an "instinctive" behavior which 2)
serves a dual adaptive function of choosing an
appropriate and safe environment and coordinates
the period of sleep in the daily cycle of
instinctive behavior; there follows a 3) necessary
set of inhibitory activities which 4) permits recovery or restoration of the "plastic" synapses.
Pavlov typically combined his inhibitory theory
with a recovery consequence: "During the period
when the cells are in a state of inhibition...the
cortical elements recover their normal state." And
Claparede added to his protective statement: "The
importance of the restorative state has been
proved..." Both Webb and Meddis flirt with instincts
and biorhythm conceptualizations.
    Allison and Van Twyver, in their evolutionary
considerations, linked the energy conservation and
ecological theories. After their development of
the energy conservation role of sleep they go on:
"...There are several factors that determine how
much a particular species needs to sleep, but
perhaps the clearest is the predator/prey relationship (and) the essential differences between good
sleepers and poor sleepers depends upon the securi-
tyof the animals sleeping arrangement" (Allison &
Van Twyver, 1970, p. 63). Recently Allison and
Chichetti performed a correlational analysis of SWS
and "activated sleep" (REM) and both constitutional
(body weight and brain weight) and ecological
variables (ratings of danger, predation and "sleep
exposure") (Allison & Chichetti, 1976). They found
that body weight and "danger" accounted for 58% of
the SWS and cautiously noted while the high negative correlation between body weight (hence metabolism) and SWS may be interpreted as terms of
"enforcing rest and hence conserving energy" that
the large species included were herbivores "which
presumably must spend large amounts of time
foraging" and were also "subject to heavy predation."

A CHOICE AMONG THEORIES?

Our review has led us into new problems.
Rather than finding ourselves midst a whirl of
incoordinate data points without thoughts of their
meanings we are faced with variety of entangled
organizing presumptions about the underlying
purposes of sleep.

In the face of these dissonances there is certainly evoked a tendency to say "Enough of this
idle speculation. Let us return to collecting
our facts." Fortunately, the power of this review
and the nature of speculative man makes this an
unlikely alternative. The heuristic value, indeed
the necessity, of theorizing is too well established in the scientific enterprise to favor such a
proposal.

A more useful alternative to abandonment,
however, would be a choice among theories. This
could concentrate our efforts in gathering facts,
testing our hypotheses, extending our reasonings
and presenting a harmonious set of explanations to
others. Unfortunately, such an alternative is not
available to us. Two minimum requirements for an
evaluation of the adequacy of a theory are: 1) it
is sufficiently articulated to permit precise
predictions and 2) the facts are available to test
the predictions. While some limited effort has
been made toward prediction, our theories to date
have been generally post hoc attempts to coordinate
selected sets of sleep phenomena and data. Further
our data have been often barely sufficient to argue
from (Webb, 1974b). In such a state of affairs one
can only make choices on the grounds on which the
theories are propounded: argument or criticism.
The limitations of this method of choice have been
well stated (Dallenbach, 1953):

"Indeed, though I have searched through the
history of our science (psychology) for a theory
that gave way to criticism and been unable to find
one... Theories do not succumb to abstract argumen-
tation... they pass from the scientific stage not
because they have been discredited but because they
have been superceded or bypassed-pushed off the
stage and replaced with other theories."

THE FUTURE OF THEORIES

As noted, it is unlikely that our speculation about the "why" of sleep will cease. Some of the current positions will continue to be elaborated upon, sharpened and modified by the search for data relevant to their predictions and prejudices. Hopefully, they will be extended to incorporate broader aspects of the sleep phenomena.

But in these future searches I would adjure that we recognize and we maintain a substantive aspect that has been introduced into our theorizing by the ecological theories. This approach is fundamentally different from the classical physical science model which is the format of most research including sleep research and is the fundament of the older theories. This classical model is oriented toward the search for physical and bio-chemical mechanisms that serve as proximal antecedants to direct consequence. The focus is on "how" an event is organized. In contrast the ethological approach places emphasis on questions of function or purpose of events or "why". This theorizing tends to be behaviorly, contextually, and consequence oriented. It follows Tinbergen's urgings to direct our efforts to understanding "the effects of behavior; of the ways in which it influences the survival of the species (and) to understand the state of adaptedness and the process of evolutionary adaptation" (Tinbergen, 1969, p.ix).

The contrast between these approaches was noted in a comparison of an ethological theory with the restorative theories (Webb, 1975, p. 162). The first position sees sleep occurring "...because the appropriate behavior behavior is elicited by the circumstances of the surroundings and the time "while the later...sees sleep as a response to some increasing build up of noxious states or as a deprivation condition requiring sleep in order to restore..." In the first model one seeks the causes in the environment, while in the latter the cause lies within the organism.

This, of course, is not a plea that we abandon our inquiries into the "mechanisms" or "efficient causes" of sleep. These are not incompatible but rather are additive approaches. Rather it seeks an emphasis and a continuing interest in placing our concepts within the contextual settings of the organisms in both an evolutionary and contemporary sense.

Above all our hope for the future of theories would be that, as facts cumulate and thoughts sharpen, our theories will take a deductive form which will permit us to predict such variables as sleep onset, amounts, placement and sleep terminationboth across and within species. That will be the ultimate testing ground of all our present intuitions.

FUNCTION AND CLINICAL IMPLICATIONS

There has been an effort in this review to consider the present status of existant theories dispassionately. In this conclusive section, I select the position with which I am identified and most familiar and try to spell out some of the clinical implications of the functions of sleep theories. Specifically, I refer to an ethological position as outlined in four earlier statements (Webb, 1971, 1974a, 1974b, 1975).

This conceptualization views the "function" of sleep as an adaptive one; "one of many complicated systems of mechanisms that protect it against the influences of the environment and enables it to maintain itself as a living organism." Such systems have certain general characteristics which I believe describe sleep as well as tell us much about its particular functions:

1)   Sleep is unlearned, inherent or innate.

2)   Sleep displays systemic developmental patterns.

3)   Sleep is species specific but has a range of intraspecies variations.

4)   Sleep displays adaptive qualities by being both flexible and having boundary conditions.

I believe these qualities to be descriptive of sleep. It is a fortunate endowment given each passing generation and each person within that generation. It shows remarkably certain developmental patterns which parents would do well to nurture rather than struggle with. There are important individual variation within the ordered

and lawful properties within each species.   Impor-
tantly sleep is adaptive in each environment.   Again
it permits us necessary variations to respond to
danger or needs, stands sturdily in the face of
minor variations, exacts its presence when we extend
unhealthily beyond its boundary conditions.

Beyond being descriptive of sleep as I "understand" it, the implications to this adaptive position, I feel, are yet more profound.   I am again
indebted to Tinbergen for a clarifying statement
(1969, p. x):

"...the developments of physics and chemistry
have shown (that) a knowledge of causes provides us
with the power to manipulate events and 'bully them
into subservience' ...Man, particularly Urban man,
is inclined even in his biological studies to ape
physics, and so to contribute to the satisfaction
of his urge to conquer nature...we have changed our
environment in which the behavior was molded and,
as a consequence, misfires."

My position views sleep as a process which
evolved to aid us to adapt our behavior to an environment of eons ago.   The sleep of Babylon is the
sleep of today.   For those times and places it functioned effectively as a biological system.   But,
modern times have brought the Edison Age of electric
lights and is abolishing the natural rhythm of
night and day, the jet aircraft tosses sleep across
multiply time zones, and drugs have given promises
of bending sleep to our momentary demands.   Perva-
sively, we raise our strident cries and push our
self-centered demands that sleep be subservient to
our whimsy, bend to our needs, pressures and
terrors.   We ominously move toward viewing our
failures of sleep to be "illnesses" to be "cured."

My view point is to the contrary.   In a reasonably natural and stable environment sleep will serve
its function as a silent and well-trained servant.
It is rather our "misbehaviors" in relation to
sleep, goaded by a changed environment and a
thoroughly anthropomorphic arrogance about "nature",
which "fails" sleep as it is pushed beyond its
natural limits.   From my perspective, anchored in
my adaptive theory of sleep, we must rather than
learn the proximal causes of sleep, learn the laws
of sleep.   In turn we must teach ourselves to act
in accord with these laws.   I agree with Francis
Bacon of 500 years ago: "Nature cannot be command-
ed except by being obeyed."

FOOTNOTE

[1]The term theory is used here in its weakest
sense of a "tentative explanation of a phenomenon".

ACKNOWLEDGMENT

The support of NIA Grant AG/MH 00805-01 is
gratefully acknowledged.

REFERENCES

Adams, K. and Oswald, I. Why sleep is a time of
    greater net protein synthesis, (Abstract),
    Association for the Psychophysiological Study
    of Sleep, 1976.

Allison, T. and Van Twyver, H. The evolution of
    sleep. Natural History, 79: 56-65, 1970.

Allison, T. and Chichetti, D. Sleep in Mammals:
    Ecological and Constitutional correlates.
    Science, 194: 732-734, 1976.

Aristotle. De Somnis. In W. Ross (Ed.), DeAnima.
    Oxford: Clarendon Press, 1951.

Berger, R. J. Bioenergetic functions of sleep
    and activity of rhythms and their possible
    relevance to aging. Proceedings of the
    Federation of American Society for Experi-
    mental Biology, 34: 97-102, 1975.

Claparede, E. Esquisse d'une theorie biologique
    du Sommeil. Archives of Psychology, 4:
    245-349, 1905.

Dallenbach, K. The place of theory in science.
    Psychological Review, 60: 33-69, 1953.

Duhem, Pierre. The Aim and Structure of Physical
    Theory (trans. Weiner), Princeton, 1954,
    (First published as La Theorie Physique,
    Paris, 1914).

Fishbein, W. and Gutwein, B. Paradoxical sleep
and memory storage processes. Behavioral
Biology, 19: 425-464, 1977.

Greenberg, R. and Pearlman, C. A. Cutting the
REM nerve: An approach to the adaptive role
of REM sleep. Perspectives in Biology and
Medicine, Summer, 513-521, 1974.

Hartmann, E. The Functions of Sleep. New Haven:
Yale University Press, 1973.

Hess, W. R. The diencephalic sleep centre. In
J. Delafresnaye (Ed.), Brain Mechanisms and
Consciousness. Springfield: Thomas, 1954.

Jouvet, M. Neurophysiology of the states of sleep.
Physiological Reviews, 47: 117-193, 1967.

Kleitman, N. Sleep and Wakefulness (2nd ed.).
Chicago: University of Chicago Press, 1963.

McGinty, D. J. Encephalization and the neural
control of behavior. In. M.B. Sterman, D.J.
McGinty and A. M. Adinolfi (Eds.), Brain
Development and Behavior. New York: Academic
Press, 1971.

McGinty, J. J., Harper, T. M. and Fairbanks, M. K.
Neuronal Unit Activity and the Control of
Sleep States. In E. Weitzman (Ed.), Advances
in Sleep Research (Vol. I). New York:
Spectrum Publications, 1974.

Meddis, R. The function of sleep. Animal Behavior,
23: 676-691, 1975.

Meddis, R. The Sleep Instinct. London: Routledge
and Kegan Paul, 1977.

Moruzzi, G. The functional significance of sleep
with particular regard to the brain mechanisms
underlying consciousness. In. J. C. Eccles
(Ed.), Brain and Conscious Experience. New
York: Springer, 1966.

Moruzzi, G.   The sleep waking cycle.   Erbenisse du
     Physiologie, 64: 1-165, 1972.

Moruzzi, G. and Magoun, H. W.   Brain stem reticular
     formation and the activation of the EEG.
     Electroencephalography and Clinical Neuro-
     physiology, I, 455-473, 1949.

Oswald, I.   Sleep the great restorer.   New
     Scientist, 46: 170-172, 1970.

Oswald, I.   Sleep.   Harmondsworth, Middlesex:
     Penguin Books, 1974.

Pavlov, I. P.   Conditioned Reflexes.   Oxford:
     Oxford Press, 1927.

Snyder, F.   Toward an evolutionary theory of dream-
     ing.   American Journal of Psychiatry, 123:
     121-134, 1962.

Snyder, F.   Evolutionary theories of sleep.   What,
     Which, Whether.   In M. Chase (Ed.), The
     Sleeping Brain.   Los Angeles: Brain Informa-
     tion Service, 1972.

Tinbergen, N.   The Study of Instinct.   New York:
     Oxford Press, 1969.

Webb, W. B.   Sleep: An Experimental Analysis.
     New York: MacMillan, 1968.

Webb, W. B.   Sleep as a biorhythm.   In P.
     Colóquhoun (Ed.), Biological Rhythms and
     Human Performance.   London: Academic Press,
     1971.

Webb, W. B.   Sleep: An Active Process.   Glenview:
     Scott, Foresman, 1973.

Webb, W. B.   Sleep as an adaptive response.
     Perceptual and Motor Skills, 38: 1023-1027,
     1974a.

Webb, W. B.   The adaptive functions of sleep
     patterns.   In P. Levin and W. P. Koella (Eds.),
     Sleep.   Basel: Karger, 1974b.

Webb, W. B. Sleep: The Gentle Tyrant. Englewood Cliffs: Prentice-Hall, 1975.

Williams, H. L., Holloway, F. and Griffiths, W. Physiological Psychology: Sleep. American Review of Psychology, 24: 279-305, 1973.

Zepelin, H. and Rechtshaffen, A. Mammalian Sleep, Longevity, and Energy Metabolism. Brain, Behavior and Evolution, 10: 425, 1974.

RETICULAR FORMATION ACTIVITY AND REM SLEEP

JEROME M. SIEGEL

Neurophysiology Research
Sepulveda Veterans Administration Hospital
Sepulveda, California

and

Brain Research Institute
University of California
Los Angeles, California

It is unlikely that we will be able to understand the function of REM sleep until we know what brain areas generate and control it. Many groups of investigators have attempted to locate the brain structures responsible for this state. The conclusions of these investigations have been thrown into increasing doubt by recent developments which I will attempt to review.

TRANSECTION AND LESION DATA

General Considerations

The classical approach to analyzing the operation of biological systems has been to remove portions of the system and determine what functions are lost. The limitations of this procedure are often not adequately considered. REM sleep is a fragile state. It is easily disrupted by a variety of non-specific factors. Therefore, the significance of a reduction or loss of REM sleep after destruction of brainstem areas must be carefully assessed.

Studies of sleep utilizing brainstem transections or lesions repeatedly note a variety of problems with the general health of the animal including skin ulcerations, hematuria, hypoglycemia, uremia, hyperkalemia, cardiac arrhythmias, vomiting, hyperthermia, hypothermia, aphagia and adipsia, and absence of spontaneous micturition and defecation (Villablanca, 1966; Hobson, 1965; Bard and

Copyright © 1979 by Academic Press, Inc.
All rights of reproduction in any form reserved.
ISBN 0-12-222340-3

Macht, 1958; Jouvet, 1962; Roussel et al., 1976;
Jones et al., 1977). Apneusis and reductions in
respiratory rate severe enough to produce EEG
disturbances can result from damage in the vicinity
of the locus coeruleus (Jones et al., 1977). Most
preparations with radical brainstem lesions do not
survive the initial surgery, and those which do
require constant care to prevent death. In short,
most of these preparations are extremely ill and
are in an unstable physiological state.

Transections and lesions disrupt blood circulation through adjacent brain areas. The resulting ischemia extends the inactivated region for
unknown distances. Discharge in the cut ends of
axons, and swelling of tissues adjacent to the
lesion will contribute to disruption of remaining
tissues.

Lesions of the pontine tegmentum can disrupt
the mechanisms which produce motor inhibition in
REM sleep. This produces the syndrome of REM
sleep without atonia, in which the cat appears to
act out a dream (Jouvet and Delorme, 1965). Often
this motor behavior arouses the animal from sleep
during the SWS-REM sleep transitional state or in
the initial seconds of REM sleep (Henley and
Morrison, 1974). It has been hypothesized by
Henley and Morrison that this motor disturbance
may, in its early stages, selectively reduce or
eliminate REM sleep. This hypothesis is supported
by descriptions of cats without REM sleep after
locus coeruleus lesions. These cats typically
end a slow wave sleep (SWS) period with an abrupt
hyperextension of the neck at the time of arousal
(Jouvet and Delorme, 1965).

Neurological shock resulting from the interruption of ascending and descending pathways can lead
to a disruption of distant systems. This phenomenon has been most thoroughly studied in the spinal
cord (Sherrington, 1947). After section between
the cord and medulla, functions which are known to
be organized in the cord are lost as a result of
the disconnection of higher centers. Some functions
recover if animals survive for long enough periods,
but many are permanently disturbed. Similar phenomena occur at other levels of the neuraxis (e.g.
Sprague, 1966). Thus, the loss of REM sleep after
brain transections or lesions cannot be interpreted

as definitive proof that a REM sleep "center" has
been destroyed. This is particularly true in
light of the short survival time of many critically
important preparations (Jouvet, 1962).

Many studies have shown that lesions and transections in infant animals result in far less loss
of function than similar procedures in adult animals. Immediately after surgery, behavioral capabilities can be demonstrated in the truncated
infant nervous system that were unsuspected in
studies on adult animals (Bignall and Schramm,
1974). However, this procedure has not been
adequately applied to studies of REM sleep.

Lesions that are slowly created, by successive
enlargements in 2 or 3 separate procedures produce
far less shock to surrounding tissues than single
stage lesions (Rosner, 1970). However, lesion
studies of REM sleep mechanisms have typically employed lesions or transections carried out in a
single stage. This would tend to underestimate
the capabilities of remaining brain structures.

In summary, there are a variety of factors
which can account for the loss of neural function
after brainstem transections or lesions. It is
unlikely that there was ever any strong selective
pressure for neural circuitry to evolve to function
normally after brainstem transection. When one
considers the number of ascending and descending
tracts in the brainstem and the infinite anatomical
and physiological complexity of this area it is
remarkable that any behavioral functions survive
extensive brainstem lesions. Therefore, the loss
of REM sleep after transection or lesion cannot be
viewed as definitive evidence for the localization
of a REM sleep center. However, the presence of
REM sleep after such lesions does prove that the
ablated structures are not essential, although they
may of course contribute to normal REM sleep (e.g.
Gadea-Ciria, 1976). If, in the evaluation of
transection and lesion data, one takes this approach
of looking at those lesions which allow REM sleep
rather than looking at those which prevent it, one
is led to several novel conclusions.

Transection Data

One of the earliest studies of the behavior
of chronically maintained decerebrated cats was
performed by Bard and Macht (1958) (Fig. 1A). In
1958, before the existance of desynchronized sleep

in cats was generally known, and prior to the discovery that REM sleep was accompanied by loss of
motor tone, they pointed out that sleep occurred
in cats decerebrated at pontine or ponto-mesence-
phalic levels and that it was often accompanied by
a loss of motor tone. These observations were
extended by Jouvet (1962) with the polygraphic
recording of EEG and neck muscle tone, and the
observation of rapid eye movements and myosis
(Fig. 1A and B). Jouvet also established that the
cerebellum was not necessary for REM sleep (1962).
These observations have been repeatedly confirmed
(Hobson, 1965; Villablanca, 1966) and it has been
established that these preparations exhibit all of
the brainstem components of REM sleep, although in
reduced amounts. Furthermore, it has been shown
that severing the spinal cord at the C1 level
(Fig. 1D) does not prevent REM sleep although, like
pontine transections, it reduces REM sleep time
(Adey et al., 1968; Puizillout et al., 1974).
Certain spinal areas may, however, contribute to
the atonia of REM sleep (Morrison and Bowker, 1971).

This evidence demonstrating the survival of
REM sleep after transections clearly proves that
the brainstem, below the level of the pons and
above the spinal cord, is sufficient for the occurrence of the REM sleep state. Jouvet (1962) attempted to further localize the REM sleep center with
the use of a retropontine transection (Fig. 1C).
Just 2 cats survived this transection and then for
a duration of only 7 days. Neither cat showed
muscle atonia. This was interpreted as indicating
that the REM sleep generating mechanism was above
the cut. However, bearing in mind the many explanations of the loss of function after brain transection just discussed and particularly the fact
that small pontine lesions can produce a loss of
REM sleep atonia without preventing REM sleep
(Henley and Morrison, 1974), this negative evidence
cannot be regarded as definitive. The loss of REM
sleep may have resulted from the behavioral and
physiological abnormalities caused by the transection and not by the removal of a REM sleep
"center".

Jouvet also identified a "difficult to inter-
pret" state in brain systems anterior to the retropontine transection. This state consisted of
cortical desynchrony and myosis, during which no

visual tracking occurred. It was speculated that
this state might be a form of REM sleep generated
by a pontine center. There are many interpretations of this phenomenon that do not require postulating that this state is a form of REM sleep.
For example, this might represent an abnormal waking
condition. Indeed, Jouvet does not claim to have
demonstrated the identity of this state with REM
sleep. Yet this is the crucial piece of positive
evidence supporting the hypothesis that the pons
contains the generator neurons for REM sleep. Therefore, if one conservatively evaluates the transection
data, one is forced to conclude that the system generating REM sleep may be located anywhere between
the cervical spinal cord and the anterior pons. It
is true, however, that PGO (pontine-geniculate-
occipital) spikes, a phenomenon common to REM sleep,
waking, (Bowker and Morrison, 1976) and drug induced
states, can be generated by the isolated pons
(Laurent et al., 1974).

Lesion Data

Several series of lesion studies have been
performed in order to further localize the areas
responsible for REM sleep. While it has been
possible to prevent REM sleep by brainstem lesions,
the findings have not been consistent.
Carli and Zanchetti (1965), in an extensive
series of studies in 40 cats identified the nucleus
reticularis pontis oralis (RPO) as the structure
whose destruction was most consistently correlated
with REM sleep suppression. They specifically rule
out the locus coeruleus and sub coeruleus as essential for REM sleep, since extensive lesions in
these areas were not correlated with great reductions in REM sleep time.
Jouvet in his initial studies (1962) identified the nucleus reticularis pontis caudalis (RPC)
as the critical structure for REM sleep. This
nucleus, as defined by Jouvet, overlaps somewhat
with Carli and Zanchetti's definition of RPO.
However, further studies by Jouvet's group pointed
to the locus coeruleus not the RPC as the crucial
structure (Jouvet, 1972; Roussel et al., 1976).
It was also found that lesions restricted to caudal
locus coeruleus produced REM sleep without atonia
(Jouvet and Delorme, 1965). Recently, Jones et al.
(1977) have contended that locus coeruleus lesions

produce only a loss of the atonia of REM sleep. In
agreement with Carli and Zanchetti (1965), they
conclude that REM sleep remains after destruction
of locus coeruleus. Similarly, locus coeruleus
lesions in kittens did not disrupt REM sleep
(Adrien, 1975).

Henley and Morrison (1974) have demonstrated
that locus coeruleus lesions are not even required
to produce the syndrome of REM sleep without atonia.
They produced REM sleep without atonia with small
lesions in the region of RPO. They suggest that
Carli and Zanchetti's (1965) finding of a loss of
REM sleep after RPO lesions may have resulted from
their not detecting REM sleep periods without atonia
However, Carli and Zanchetti were aware of the
"hallucinating" episodes previously reported and
specifically mention that they did not observe this
phenomenon. They also recorded pontine PGO spikes
which would have helped locate such episodes.

It is by no means certain that further studies
of lesions disrupting REM sleep will clarify the
issue of the anatomical location of structures
generating it. The principal histological differences between lesions disrupting REM sleep and
those sparing it, is the size of the lesions, i.e.,
Jouvet et al.'s locus coeruleus lesions and Carli
and Zanchetti's RPO lesions which eliminated REM
sleep signs were larger than the lesions created by
Jones et al.(1977) and Henley and Morrison (1974)
which did not abolish REM sleep. Carli and
Zanchetti (1965) reported that moderate sized lesions of either the medial RPO or the lateral RPO
do not abolish REM sleep, while larger lesions
destroying both these areas do. This strengthens
the argument that nonspecific effects such as
trauma, imbalances of neural circuits, or shock in
deafferented systems, are the likely explanation of
REM sleep loss after these brainstem lesions.

Even if a small, specific region whose destruction eliminated REM sleep could be identified,
this would not prove that it was the REM sleep
"center." This can be illustrated by the finding
of McGinty and Sterman (1968) that lesions of the
basal forebrain region (Fig. 1) totally eliminated
REM sleep for periods of several weeks; this despite the fact that the basal forebrain is not
required for REM sleep, since it is well anterior

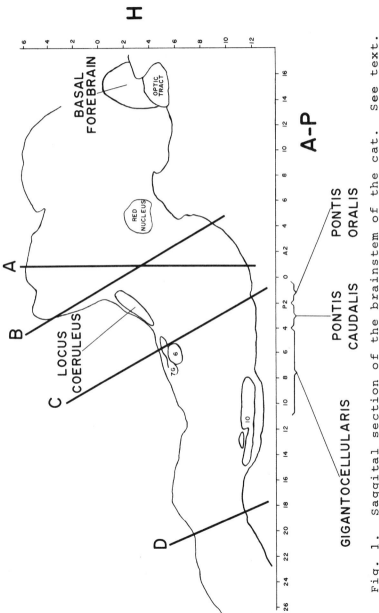

Fig. 1. Saggital section of the brainstem of the cat. See text.

to the transections performed by Bard and Macht
(1958) and Jouvet (1962) which allowed REM sleep.
Lesions of more caudal structures might well
produce REM sleep suppressions equal to or greater
than those resulting from basal forebrain lesions,
even if these areas were not part of the executive
mechanisms for REM sleep.

In summary: 1) Transection data clearly
localize REM sleep generating mechanisms to the
brainstem region lying between the spinal cord and
the anterior pons. 2) The main evidence localizing
REM sleep generating mechanisms to specific areas
within the brainstem is based on the loss of REM
sleep after lesions. Nonspecific factors may be
responsible for this loss of function. 3) Therefore, on the basis of lesion and transection evidence we cannot confidently localize REM sleep
generating mechanisms to any particular nucleus
within the brainstem.

UNIT RECORDING DATA

General Considerations

Another method for localizing the cell groups
generating REM sleep is the recording of the activity of brainstem units during the sleep cycle.
This approach allows observation of the normal
functioning of single cells. To the extent that
cells in a given cytological area show similar
types of activity changes across the sleep cycle,
the discharge patterns of large brainstem areas
can be determined.

The presence of cell discharge correlated
with REM sleep does not prove that a cell group
is necessary or even important in REM sleep generation. However, a cell group whose activity is
found not to relate closely to REM sleep is unlikely
to have an important role in its control.

Most brain neurons show substantial increases
in their activity during REM sleep. Therefore,
cell discharge must be carefully examined in a
variety of behavioral situations to determine
whether or not a relationship to REM is an epiphe-
nomenon related to one of the many physiological
processes influenced by REM sleep. Before a cell
group can be accepted as forming the "executive"

mechanism of REM sleep, it must be shown to relate to the complex of physiological events that
identify the REM sleep state. If this requirement is not fulfilled we are forced to accept the
simplest plausible explanation of changes in activity, i.e., that the cell group is involved in
the regulation of posture, phasic motor activity,
eye movement, EEG activation, etc.

It must then be shown that procedures which
selectively increase discharge in this cell group
(such as electrical or neurochemical stimulation)
increase REM sleep duration or intensity (assuming
the cells are facilitatory to REM sleep) while
procedures that decrease activity in these cell
groups (such as lesion or neurochemical inactiva-
tion) decrease REM sleep duration or intensity.
Nonspecific effects of the procedures used to
change cell discharge rates must be experimentally determined.

We have been engaged in studies of units in
the medial pontobulbar reticular formation. One
motive for studying this region is that it includes the areas that several of the previously
discussed lesion studies indicated might be required for REM sleep.

A second motive for studying this region is
that it is known to have widespread connections
with a variety of brain areas. Regardless of
whether it has an executive role in the control
of REM sleep, it is hard to imagine any REM sleep
generating system that would not employ elements
of the medial reticular formation as a pathway to
convey physiological changes throughout the central
nervous system.

A third reason for studying this structure in
relation to sleep is that it has been so thoroughly studied from several other perspectives. Indeed,
with the possible exception of the visual cortex,
the mammalian reticular formation has probably
been more intensively studied than any other brain
structure. However, with only a few exceptions,
studies of unit discharge in reticular formation
cells have been carried out in paralyzed, anesthe-
tized or restrained animals. Thus, an understanding of the functional significance of activity in these cells, based on observations in a
variety of behavioral situations, has not been
possible. Therefore, we have been recording

activity in these cells in unrestrained cats and
observing the behavioral correlates of their discharge during both sleep and waking.

Pontine Nucleus Gigantocellularis

The first target of investigation was the
pontine nucleus gigantocellularis, or FTG (gigantocellular tegmental field) in Bermans (1968) terminology. This nucleus occupies a large portion
of the brainstem reticular formation. A total of
85 units has been recorded in this area (Siegel
et al., 1977).

Three types of gigantocellularis units could
be distinguished on the basis of discharge patterns
during the sleep-waking cycle. Type one cells
had no spontaneous activity during quiet waking,
SWS or REM sleep (Fig. 2). They discharged in
association with movements and were otherwise
silent. These cells are unique in being the only
group of brain cells observed which normally show
no activity during either REM sleep or SWS. In a
quiet, waking animal these cells can be completely silent for periods of up to 40 minutes or
more (Siegel and McGinty, 1976). Twenty-eight
percent of pontine gigantocellularis cells were
of this type.

The second cell type had relatively high
levels of tonic activity in both waking and sleep
(Fig. 3). Its defining characteristic was a discharge rate greater than 4 spikes/second. These
cells showed a relatively small rate increase
during the SWS-REM sleep transition. Fifteen percent of gigantocellularis cells were of this type.

The third cell type had an intermediate level
of spontaneous discharge in quiet waking and slow
wave sleep (Fig. 4). However, it discharged in
bursts during both waking movements and REM sleep.
Fifty-seven percent of gigantocellularis cells
were of this type.

Considering the group of pontine gigantocellularis cells as a whole there was a strong,
highly significant positive correlation between a
neuron's maximum waking discharge rate and its
average or maximum REM sleep rate, i.e., neurons
with high REM sleep rates also had high rates
during waking. We saw no gigantocellularis cells

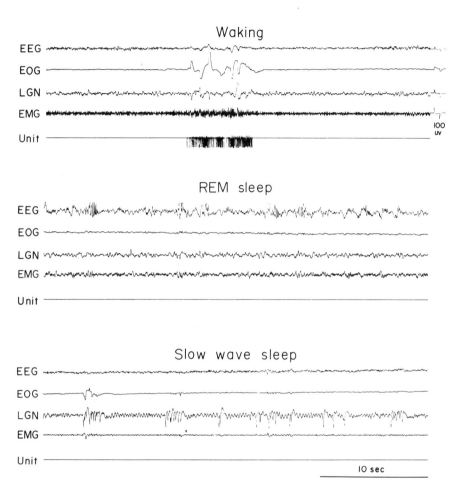

Fig. 2. A type 1 pontine gigantocellularis neuron. Labels for this and succeeding figures: EEG - sensorimotor electoencephalogram; EOG - electrooculogram; LGN - lateral geniculate nucleus; EMG - dorsal neck muscle electromyogram. (From *Experimental Neurology* 56: 553-573, 1977).

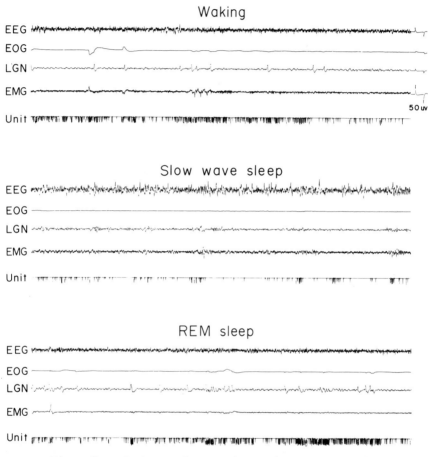

Fig. 3. A type 2 pontine gigantocellularis
neuron. (From Experimental Neurology 56: 553-
573, 1977).

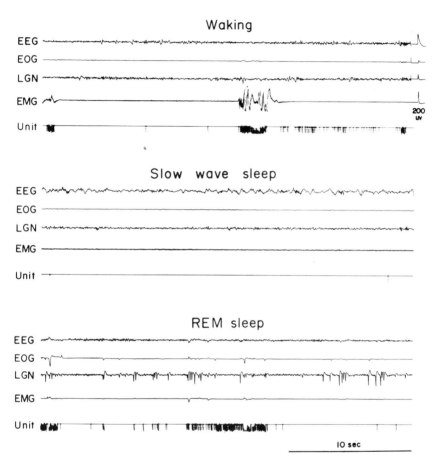

Fig. 4. A type 3 pontine gigantocellularis neuron. (From Experimental Neurology 56: 553-573, 1977).

which discharged selectively in REM sleep. All
gigantocellularis cells exceeded their mean REM
sleep discharge rates during waking movement
(Siegel et al., 1977).

We have systematically observed the behavioral correlates of waking discharge in these cells
(Siegel and McGinty, 1977). Cells were found to
relate to specific movements of either the head
and neck, ear, forepaw, scapula, or tongue.

Many of these cells also responded to applied
sensory stimuli (Fig. 5). However, the responses
to applied stimuli were generally brief and
habituated rapidly. In this respect, gigantocellularis discharge appears to correlate with the brief
motor activity of the startle response. Only when
sustained movements were evoked by stimuli did
sustained gigantocellularis discharge occur.

In 15 cells the sensory stimuli which were
found to evoke unit activity were systematically
eliminated or attenuated. Vestibular stimuli,
which were the best stimuli for most cells, were
eliminated by an atraumatic head restraint system.
Somatic stimuli were eliminated by local anesthesia
of identified receptive fields. Auditory stimuli
were attenuated by occluding the ear canals with
cotton impregnated with wax. Visual stimuli were
eliminated by placing the cat in a light tight box.
In no case did this stimulus reduction procedure
greatly reduce or eliminate cell discharge. In
most instances unit activity increased. This increase in firing was correlated with phasic bursts
of EMG activity (Fig. 6). This experiment demonstrates that gigantocellularis discharge is more
closely related to motor output than it is to
sensory input.

If restraint continued for more than 3-5
minutes both motor activity and correlated gigantocellularis discharge decreased (Fig. 7). A cat
which has previously experienced restraint and is
undisturbed will show very little struggling and
hence virtually no unit discharge during waking.
Therefore, estimates of waking discharge rates in
such preparations will greatly underestimate the
"average" waking rate. As a consequence, the discharge in these cells will appear to be selective
for REM sleep. Previous studies by Hobson and
McCarley and their co-workers (McCarley and Hobson,
1971; Hobson et al., 1974) which found that

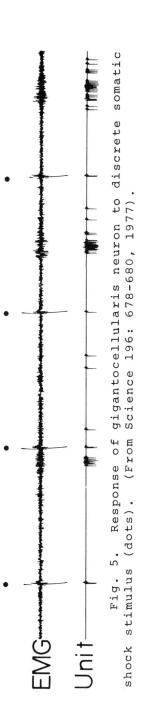

Fig. 5. Response of gigantocellularis neuron to discrete somatic shock stimulus (dots). (From Science 196: 678-680, 1977).

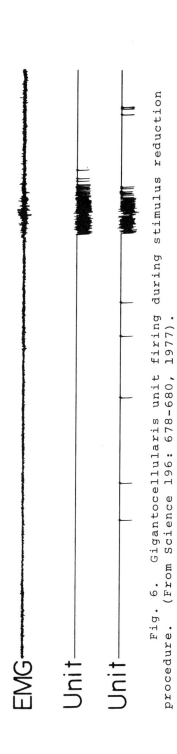

Fig. 6. Gigantocellularis unit firing during stimulus reduction procedure. (From Science 196: 678-680, 1977).

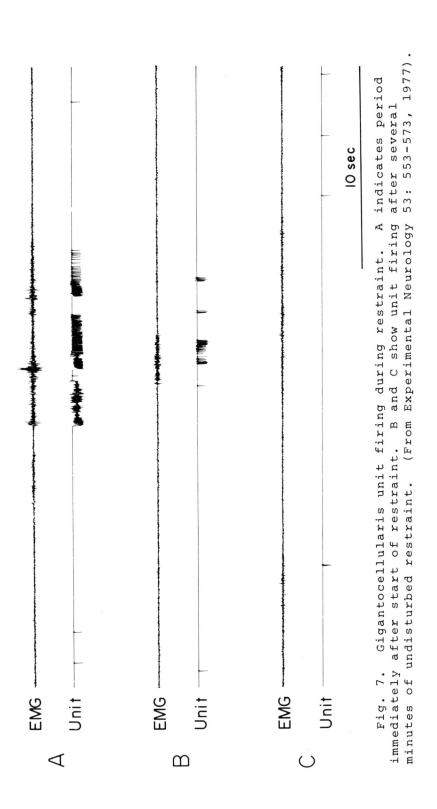

Fig. 7. Gigantocellularis unit firing during restraint. A indicates period immediately after start of restraint. B and C show unit firing after several minutes of undisturbed restraint. (From Experimental Neurology 53: 553-573, 1977).

gigantocellularis cells had discharge selective for
REM sleep used cats adapted to head restraint.
Similarly, studies by Pompeiano and Hoshino
(Pompeiano and Hoshino, 1976a; Hoshino and
Pompeiano, 1976) which reported that gigantocellu-
laris cells discharge selectively during cataplec-
tic episodes induced by an anticholinesterase, used
cats which were immobilized by decerebration.

Most gigantocellularis cells fired rhythmical-
ly during some grooming periods (Fig. 8). This
illustrates several important points about these
cells. 1) It has been reported that these cells
habituate to repetitive sensory stimulation (e.g.,
Scheibel and Scheibel, 1965; Peterson et al., 1976),
but during the rhythmic motor activity of grooming
no habituation occurs. We also find that units do
not habituate to sensory stimuli which repeatedly
evoke specific movements. 2) During grooming, reciprocal discharge can be seen in pairs of gigantocellularis cells which are correlated with different movements. This sort of discharge pattern is
incompatible with the concept that these cells are
related to nonspecific arousal. 3) The high discharge rate during spontaneous behaviors demonstrates that painful stimuli are not required to acti-
vate these cells (e.g., Casey, 1969).

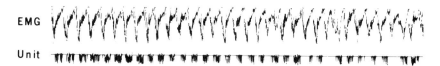

EMG

Unit

Fig. 8. Gigantocellularis unit discharge
during grooming. (From Science 196: 678-680, 1977).

Our behavioral evidence leads to the conclusion that <u>discharge in gigantocellularis cells is
a correlate of motor activity</u>. Since movement is a
normal accompaniment of a variety of behavioral
processes, the motor related activity of pontine
gigantocellularis cells can explain many of their
previously reported relationships to habituation,
arousal processes and painful stimuli (Siegel and
McGinty, 1977). Their discharge in phasic bursts

during REM sleep is also consistent with this view,
since REM sleep is a time of intense motor activation. We see no cells in this area whose discharge pattern is consistent with an executive role
in REM sleep generation.

Nucleus Reticulus Pontis Oralis and Caudalis

The second portion of the medial reticular
formation investigated was the area of the nucleus
reticularis pontis oralis and caudalis. This region lies just anterior to the nucleus gigantocellularis and is the location that Carli and
Zanchetti's extensive lesion studies pinpoint as
being critical for REM sleep (1965).

Our microdrive bundles were aimed at the
center of the region identified by Carli and
Zanchetti. We have recorded a total of 22 cells
in 3 cats. Their sleep waking discharge patterns
do not differ greatly from those observed in the
gigantocellularis region. We see the same 3 cell
types (Fig. 9). Fourteen percent are type one,
50% type 2 and 36% type 3. Cells with high REM
sleep discharge rates tend to have high rates in
waking. We see no cells which discharge selectively in REM sleep.

Waking discharge relates to motor activity.
However, these cells do not relate primarily to
lateral head movements in the way that cells in the
gigantocellular nucleus do; instead, they appear to
relate to activity in trunk musculature. More of
these cells must be investigated before the nature
of movement correlations can be clearly understood.

Medullary Gigantocellular Nucleus

The third portion of the medial reticular formation investigated was the medullary portion of
the gigantocellular nucleus. This is just caudal
to, and continuous with the pontine gigantocellular
nucleus. This area overlaps a portion of the
Magoun inhibitory region (Magoun, 1944; Magoun and
Rhines, 1946). Netick, Orem and Dement (1977) recently described 6 cells found in the medullary
gigantocellular region which discharged selectively in REM sleep.

We have explored the portion of this area
between P9 and P11 in 3 cats. We see the same

WAKING

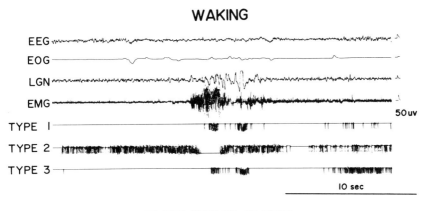

SLOW WAVE SLEEP

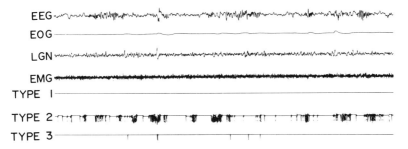

REM SLEEP

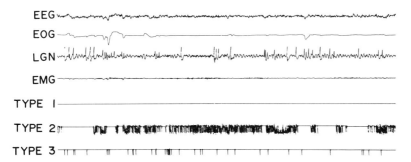

Fig. 9. Simultaneous recording of the three cell types seen in nucleus reticularis pontis caudalis and oralis area.

3 cell types in this area that we found in RPO,
RPC and in the pontine gigantocellular area. Of
the 29 cells recorded, 28% are type one, 41% type
2 and 31% type 3.

Waking discharge related to motor activity as
was the case in the more anterior regions. Several
cells in this area discharged at high rates when
the cat held particular postures. If the cat shifted into a different position, the discharge rate
was greatly reduced.

We saw no cells which discharged selectively
in REM sleep, as Netick, Orem and Dement (1977)
reported. However, 2 of the posture related cells
discharged at a low rate in quiet waking and SWS,
showed a tonic rate increase during the SWS-REM
sleep transition and maintained this rate throughout REM sleep. Therefore, the sleep and quiet
waking behavior of these cells is strikingly similar to that of the cells seen by Netick, Orem and
Dement (Fig. 10). Since these workers were recording from cats which were adapted to head restraint,
they would not have been able to observe unit activity in a variety of postures. Therefore, it
appears likely that the REM sleep selective cells
they observed are similar to the posture related
cells which we have seen. If this is the case,
then the REM sleep related acceleration can be
understood as reflecting the motor activation of
REM sleep. Just as cells which are phasically
active in waking show phasic activity in REM sleep,
these cells, which discharge tonically while
postures are maintained in waking also show tonic
REM sleep activity. It is also conceivable that
medullary REM sleep selective cells are rare and
were missed by our microelectrodes. Further investigation of this area is required.

In summary: We have explored the medial
brainstem reticular formation from H.C. coordinates
P2 to P11. We find that cells in this area are
related to motor activity in waking. During REM
sleep they show discharge patterns which resemble
their waking activity. Discharge rates in the two
states are postively correlated. These findings
suggest a role for these cells in mediating the
motor activation of both waking and sleep, but are
not consistent with an executive role for these
neurons in the generation of REM sleep.

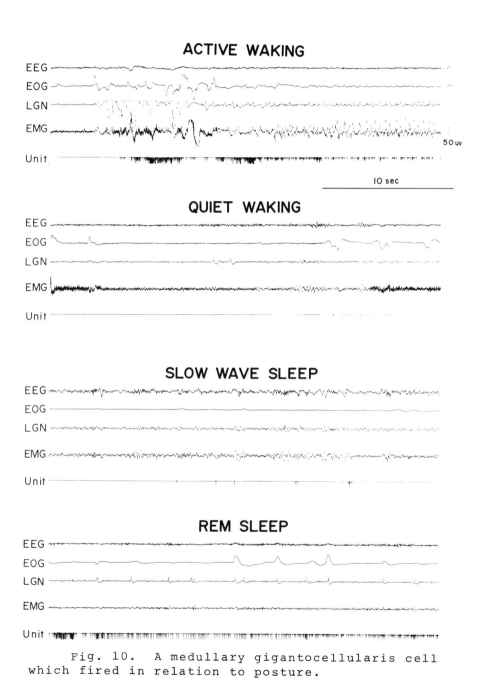

Fig. 10. A medullary gigantocellularis cell which fired in relation to posture.

DISCUSSION

     In the first portion of this presentation I
reviewed the lesion and transection evidence localizing the brain structures responsible for REM
sleep. This evidence demonstrates that the integrity of the pontomedullary brainstem is sufficient
for the periodic occurrence of REM sleep. However,
lesion evidence does not definitively localize the
region crucial for REM sleep.
     Unit recording evidence was then presented.
These studies reveal a relationship between reticular formation unit activity and movement. They
are consistent with the discharge of these cells
in REM sleep, whose most obvious behavioral manifestation is motor activation. However, this unit
data is essentially negative with respect to the
goal of anatomically localizing the neurons responsible for REM sleep. None of the 136 cells studied
discharged selectively in REM sleep. None of these
neurons appear to be REM sleep "executive" neurons.
     There are several possible explanations for
our inability to find REM sleep executive neurons
in the brainstem.
     1) There may be REM sleep executive neurons
within the medial reticular area that we have not
encountered. We did not record activity at all
lateralities and all anteroposterior levels. The
fact that medial reticular formation cells from P2
to P11 appear to be fairly homogeneous with respect
to their sleep related activity, makes it appear
unlikely that there would be a large cluster of
undiscovered REM sleep selective cells within this
area. However, if REM sleep executive cells are
relatively few in number and are not anatomically
clustered, they might have escaped detection. The
RPO, RPC and medullary gigantocellular nuclei have
not been as thoroughly explored as the pontine
gigantocellular nucleus, and are therefore promising
areas for further study.
     2) The REM executive elements may not have
been detected because they were too small for our
electrodes. While our microwire technique has been
shown capable of recording cells as small as 30μ
(McGinty and Harper, 1976), it would not resolve
extremely small neurons. However, in general, it
has been our experience that cells with small

action potentials were type 2 cells, i.e., they showed less rate increase in REM sleep than most other cells.

A related possibility is that glial elements are responsible for triggering REM sleep. Intracellular studies of glial slow potentials during sleep might shed light on their role.

3) The REM sleep executive neurons may exist in other brainstem areas. The vestibular nuclei appear to have been eliminated on the basis of both lesion and recording studies (Perenin et al., 1972; Bizzi et al., 1964; Morrison and Pompeiano, 1966) although they may affect PGO spike distribution. Similarly the midline raphe nuclei do not appear to be essential for REM sleep, although they may have important roles in the regulation of arousal and of PGO spikes (Simon et al., 1973).

Unit activity in and around the locus coeruleus has been the subject of several studies (Chu and Bloom, 1973; Pompeiano and Hoshino, 1976b; Hobson et al., 1975; Saito et al., 1977). It has been found that many of these cells show a remarkable suppression of discharge apparently specific to REM sleep. Evidence has been presented by Carli and Zanchetti (1965) and more recently by Jones et al. (1977) showing survival of REM sleep after locus coeruleus lesions. This evidence is not consistent with an executive role for these neurons in REM sleep control. If it can be confirmed that complete locus coeruleus lesions are compatible with REM sleep, then the locus coeruleus activity change in REM sleep must be understood primarily in relation to the peripheral variables of REM sleep. A major task of the future will be to establish exactly what behavioral and physiological parameters correlate with activity in these cells. A particularly interesting possibility is that these cells may relate to the control of muscle tone.

A large portion of the lateral brainstem caudal to the locus coeruleus has not been systematically explored. This area might well be important in REM sleep control.

4) It seems likely that one of the first three hypotheses is the correct one. However, we should also consider a fourth hypothesis. Briefly stated, it is that there may be no "executive neurons" for

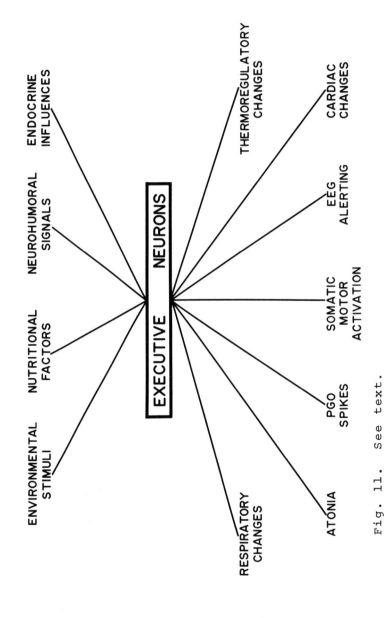

Fig. 11. See text.

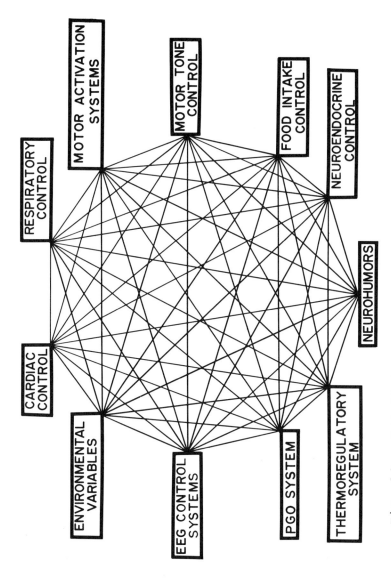

Fig. 12. See text.

REM sleep. In other words, there may be no single group of brain neurons which fulfills the requirements outlined above for "executive neurons." There are, after all, no known "executive neurons" for waking, non-REM sleep, eating, drinking or sexual behavior, although there are many neuronal groups which are known to contribute to each of these behaviors. Important behavioral processes are regulated by converging interactions from a variety of neural systems. This kind of control produces a redundancy which prevents the disruption of vital behaviors. REM sleep control can be conceptualized in a similar way, as the result of the interaction of several groups of brain neurons, with no one group having "executive" responsibility.

We can model this sort of control system and contrast it with the "executive neuron" hypothesis. The executive neuron hypothesis (Fig. 11), which is implicit in many studies attempting to anatomically localize the crucial brain substrate for REM sleep, holds that there is a group of brainstem neurons which show periodic changes in their activity. These cells receive and integrate a variety of inputs. The output of these neurons drives sensory, motor and autonomic systems, creating the behavioral and physiological manifestations of REM sleep.

In the multiple control hypothesis (Fig. 12) REM sleep results from the interaction of many groups of neurons. This figure represents some of the many systems known to influence or be influenced by REM sleep. It is not meant to be a wiring diagram of the REM sleep control mechanism, but rather to symbolically represent the extensive interconnections between these systems. The actual number of separate cell groups contributing to REM sleep control and the relative importance of individual connections between cell groups remains to be determined. Each system would have its own specific ultradian rhythmicity. According to this model, it is the network of interconnections between these systems that creates REM sleep. These interconnections synchronize and thereby enhance the amplitude of the ultradian rhythms inherent in each system. The result is the synchronous occurrence of the cyclical changes which constitute REM sleep. In this model there are no "executive neurons."

This model does not view PGO spikes as the genera-
tors of all phasic events (see Baust et al., 1972;
McGinty and Siegel, 1978, Pessah and Roffwarg,
1972).

The regions in which lesions are most effective
in disrupting REM sleep are reticular areas filled
with intersecting pathways. The REM sleep disruption caused by these lesions can be traced, according to this hypothesis primarily to the destruction of axons, not of cell bodies. The acute
effects of destruction of any single system might
be the disruption of the entire REM sleep generating network as a result of neurological shock.
However, if slowly enlarged lesions, infant animals,
and long recovery periods were employed, many of
the phenomena of REM sleep might reappear as a
result of interactions between the remaining systems
above and below the lesion site. It could even be
possible in this way to create two independent
REM sleep generation networks in the same animal.
Forebrain and spinal cord states analogous to REM
sleep might be recognized in transected nervous
systems if the proper techniques for the measurement of activity were employed.

Many physiological changes that once seemed
to be uniquely restricted to REM sleep are now
known to be controlled by systems which can operate
independently. For example, PGO spikes do not
only occur in REM sleep, but also occur in waking
(Bowker and Morrison, 1976) and transitional slow
wave sleep. Lesions in the vicinity of the
vestibular nuclei may prevent PGO spike bursts
without abolishing REM sleep. PGO spikes can
also be elicited by reserpine (Brooks and Gershon,
1972) and other drugs (McGinty and Krenek, 1974).
Under these conditions they appear and disappear
periodically in a rhythm which is independent of
REM sleep. Muscle atonia similar to that seen in
REM sleep may occur during waking, resulting in
cataplectic episodes without loss of consciousness
(Mitler and Dement, 1974; Guilleminault et al.,
1974). Conversely, REM sleep may occur without
atonia (Jouvet and Delorme, 1965). Pontine transections that permit REM sleep may prevent the EKG
irregularities that normally accompany it
(Villablanca, 1966). These syndromes can be understood as the result of the partial or complete

disconnection of individual brain circuits from
the other systems involved in REM sleep control.
The result is a weakened, but independent rhythmic
oscillation in the disconnected system. The disconnection of one component should also change the
oscillation frequency of the remainder of the
system. Lesion procedures which damage systems
participating in REM sleep are known to alter the
length of the REM sleep cycle (Jouvet, 1962).

During waking the organism's interaction with
environmental stimuli would interfere with any
synchronous oscillation in these systems. However,
during the quiescence of sleep, endogenous rhythmi-
cities would not be disrupted and would synchronize
as a result of the network of interconnections.
The result would be a strong ultradian rhythm
culminating the occurrence of the phenomena of
REM sleep.

This model is consistent with findings that
stimulation of a variety of structures including
cortex (DiPaola et al., 1965) vagal nerve
(Puizillout et al., 1974) and visual system
(Rechtschaffen et al., 1969) can induce REM sleep,
even though none of these structures are required
for REM sleep. These stimulations are maximally
effective when performed in the deeper phases of
slow wave sleep. These effects would be achieved
by entraining and intensifying the ultradian increase in unit activity that characterizes REM
sleep.

The hypothesis advanced here is that it is
the network of interconnections between neural
systems that creates REM sleep. A corollary is
that understanding of REM sleep can only be
achieved by the analysis of the periodicities of
each of the physiological systems activated during
REM sleep and of the interactions between these
systems.

This theory of multiple control sites for
REM sleep suggests a subtle change in approach to
the question of "What is the function of REM
sleep?" If one thinks of a REM sleep system as
being guided by an executive neuron or neurons, it
is only natural to search for a central "motivation"
or function of these "executives." Several hypotheses as to what <u>the</u> function of REM sleep is
have been advanced. A multiple control theory

suggests a different approach. Each subsystem contributing to REM sleep would derive different benefits from REM sleep and would exert independent influence on REM sleep parameters. This approach, therefore, emphasizes the multiple functions of REM sleep.

SUMMARY

This paper considers evidence bearing on the question of the anatomical localization of mechanisms generating REM sleep.

1) Studies of sleep states after brainstem transection demonstrate that the area lying rostral to the spinal cord and caudal to the midbrain are sufficient for the occurrence of REM sleep. Investigations further localizing the mechanisms generating REM sleep are confounded by nonspecific effects which could cause loss of REM sleep after lesions.

2) Another technique for localization of REM sleep generating mechanisms is the recording of neuronal activity. Examination of brainstem reticular formation unit activity in unrestrained animals reveals 3 cell types. Type 1 cells discharge only during waking movement periods, being silent in sleep. Type 2 cells discharge at high rates during both waking and sleep, showing a small rate increase in REM sleep and waking movement periods. Type 3 cells discharge at low rates in quiet waking and slow wave sleep, and discharge at high rates during waking movement and REM sleep. All of the cells recorded in the reticularis pontis oralis, reticularis pontis caudalis, pontine gigantocellularis and medullary gigantocellularis nuclei fall into one of these 3 categories. It is suggested that these cells may mediate the motor activation common to both waking and REM sleep. No cells with discharge selective for REM sleep were found.

3) Four hypotheses explaining why no REM sleep "executive neurons" have been observed are presented. Three hypotheses derive from the assumption that technical factors have prevented observation of these cells. The fourth hypothesis considers the possibility that REM sleep "executive" cells may not exist. The implications of this hypothesis are discussed.

REFERENCES

Adey, W. R., Bors, E. and Porter, R. W.   EEG sleep patterns after high cervical lesions in man. Archives of Neurology, 19: 377-383, 1968.

Adrien, J.   Lesions of the locus coeruleus complex and of the raphe nuclei in the newborn kitten. Sleep Research, 4: 69, 1975.

Bard, P. and Macht, M. B.   The behavior of chronically decerebrate cats.   In G. E. W. Wolstenholme and L. M. O'Conner (Eds.,) Neurological Basis of Behavior.   London, Churchill, 1958, pp. 55-75.

Baust, W., Holzbach, E. and Zechlin, O.   Phasic changes in heart rate and respiration correlated with PGO-Spike activity during REM sleep.   Pflugers Archives, 331: 113-123, 1972.

Berman, A. L.   The Brain Stem of the Cat.   Madison, Wisconsin, University of Wisconsin Press, 1968.

Bignall, K. E. and Schramm, L.   Behavior of chronically decerebrated kittens.   Experimental Neurology, 42: 519-531, 1974.

Bizzi, E., Pompeiano, O. and Somogyi, I.   Spontaneous activity of single vestibular neurons of unrestrained cats during sleep and wakefulness.   Archives italiannes de Biologie, 102: 308-330, 1964.

Bowker, R. M. and Morrison, A. R.   The startle reflex and PGO spikes.   Brain Research, 102: 185-190, 1976.

Brooks, D. C. and Gershon, M. D.   An analysis of the effect of reserpine upon ponto-geniculo-occipital wave activity in the cat.   Neuropharmacology, 11: 499-510, 1972.

Carli, G. and Zanchetti, A.   A study of pontine lesions suppressing deep sleep in the cat. Archives italiannes de Biologie, 103: 751-788, 1965.

Casey, K. L. Somatic stimuli, spinal pathways, and size of cutaneous fibers influencing unit activity in the medial medullary reticular formation. Experimental Neurology, 25: 35-56, 1969.

Chu, N. and Bloom F. E. Norepinephrine-containing neurons: Changes in spontaneous discharge patterns during sleep and waking. Science, 179: 908-910, 1973.

DiPaola, M., Rossi, G. F. and Zattoni, J. Induction of EEG desynchronized sleep by electrical stimulation of the neocortex. Archives italiannes de Biologie, 103: 818-831, 1965.

Gadea-Ciria, M. Tele-encephalic versus cerebellar control upon ponto-geniculo-occipital waves during paradoxical sleep in the cat. Experientia, 32: 889-890, 1976.

Guilleminault, C., Wilson, R. A. and Dement, W.C. A study on cataplexy. Archives of Neurology, 31: 255-261, 1974.

Henley, K. and Morrison, A. R. A re-evaluation of the effects of lesions of the pontine tegmentum and locus coeruleus on phenomena of paradoxical sleep in the cat. Acta Neurobiologica Experimental, 34: 215-232, 1974.

Hobson, J. A. The effects of chronic brain-stem lesions on cortical and muscular activity during sleep and waking in the cat. Electroencephalography and clinical Neurophysiology, 19: 41-62, 1965.

Hobson, J. A., McCarley, R. W., Pivik, T. and Freedman, R. Selective firing by cat pontine brain stem neurons in desynchronized sleep. Journal of Neurophysiology, 37: 497-511, 1974.

Hobson, J. A., McCarley, R. W. and Wyzinski, P. W. Sleep cycle oscillation: Reciprocal discharge by two brainstem neuronal groups. Science, 189: 55-58, 1975.

Hoshino, K. and Pompeiano, O. Selective discharge of pontine neurons during the postural atonia produced by an anticholinesterase in the decerebrate cat. Archives italiannes de Biologie, 114: 244-277, 1976.

Jones, B. E., Harper, S. T. and Halaris, A. E. Effects of locus coeruleus lesions upon cerebral monoamine content, sleep wakefulness states and the response to amphetamine in the cat. Brain Research, 124: 473-496, 1977.

Jouvet, M. Recherches sur les structures nerveuses et les mechanismes responsables des differentes phases du sommeil physiologique. Archives italiannes de Biologie, 100: 125-206, 1962.

Jouvet, M. The role of monoamines and acetylcholine-containing neurons in the regulation of the sleep-waking cycle. Ergebnisse der Physiologie, 64: 166-307, 1972.

Jouvet, M. and Delorme, F. Locus coeruleus et sommeil paradoxal. Comptes Rendus Societe de Biologie, 159: 895-899, 1965.

Laurent, J. P., Cespuglio, R. and Jouvet, M. Delimitation des voies ascendants de l'activite ponto-geniculo-occipitale chez le chat. Brain Research, 65: 29-52, 1974.

Magoun, H. W., Bulbar inhibition and facilitation of motor activity. Science, 100: 549-550, 1944.

Magoun, H. W. and Rhines, R. An inhibitory mechanism in the bulbar reticular formation. Journal of Neurophysiology, 9: 165-171, 1946.

McCarley, R. W. and Hobson, J. A. Single neuron activity in cat gigantocellular tegmental field: Selectivity of discharge in desynchronized sleep. Science, 174: 1250-1252, 1971.

McGinty, D. J. and Harper, R. M. Dorsal raphe neurons: Depression of firing during sleep in cats. Brain Research, 101: 569-575, 1976.

McGinty, D. J. and Krenck, T. REM phenomena during alpha-chloralose anesthesia in the cat. Sleep Research, 3: 61, 1974.

McGinty, D. J. and Siegel, J. M. Sleep states. In E. Satinoff and P. Teitelbaum (Eds.), Handbook of Behavioral Neurobiology: Motivation, 1978, in press.

McGinty, D. J. and Sterman, M. B. Sleep suppression after basal forebrain lesions in the cat. Science, 160: 1253-1255, 1968.

Mitler, M. and Dement, W. Cataplectic-like behavior in cats after micro-injection of carbachol in the pontine reticular formation. Brain Research, 68: 335-343, 1974.

Morrison, A. R. and Bowker, R. M. A caudal source of cervical and forelimb inhibition during sleep. Experimental Neurology, 33: 684-692, 1971.

Morrison, A. R. and Pompeiano, O. Vestibular influences during sleep. IV. Functional relations between vestibular nuclei and lateral geniculate nucleus during desynchronized sleep. Archives italiannes de Biologie, 104: 425-458, 1966.

Netick, A., Orem, J. and Dement, W. Neuronal activity specific to REM sleep and its relationship to breathing. Brain Research, 120: 197-207, 1977.

Perenin, M. T., Maeda, T. and Jeannerod, M. Are vestibular nuclei responsible for rapid eye movements of paradoxical sleep. Brain Research, 43: 617-621, 1972.

Pessah, M. A. and Roffwarg, H. P. Spontaneous middle ear muscle activity in man: A rapid eye movement sleep phenomenon. Science, 178: 773-776, 1972.

Peterson, B. W., Franck, J. I., Pitts, N. G. and
    Daunton, N. G.   Changes in responses of
    medial pontomedullary reticular neurons
    during repetitive cutaneous, vestibular,
    cortical, and tectal stimulation. Journal
    of Neurophysiology, 39: 564-581, 1976.

Pompeiano, O. and Hoshino, K.   Central control
    of posture: Reciprocal discharge by two
    pontine neuronal groups leading to suppression
    of decerebrate rigidity. Brain Research,
    116: 131-138, 1976a.

Pompeiano, O. and Hoshino, K. Tonic inhibition of
    dorsal pontine neurons during the postural
    atonia produced by an anticholinesterase in
    the decerebrate cat. Archives italiannes de
    Biologie, 114: 310-340, 1976b.

Puizillout, J. J., Ternaux, J. P., Foutz, A. S.
    and Fernandez, G.   Les stades de sommeil de
    la preparation "encephale isole." I.
    Declenchement des pointes ponto-geniculo-
    occipitales et du sommeil phasique a ondes
    lentes.   Role des noyaux du raphe.
    Electroencephalography and Clinical Neuro-
    physiology, 37: 561-576, 1974.

Rechtschaffen, A., Dates, R., Tobias, M. and
    Whitehead, W. E.   The effect of lights-off
    stimulation on the distribution of paradoxical
    sleep in the rat. Communications in Behavioral
    Biology, A3: 93-99, 1969.

Rosner, B. S.   Brain functions. Annual Review of
    Psychology, 21: 555-594, 1970.

Roussel, B., Pujol, J. F. and Jouvet, M.   Effects
    des lesions du tegmentum pontique sur les
    etats de sommeil chez le rat. Archives
    italiannes de Biologie, 114: 188-209, 1976.

Saito, H., Sakai, K. and Jouvet, M.   Discharge
    patterns of the nucleus parabrachialis
    lateralis neurons of the cat during sleep and
    waking. Brain Research, 1977, in press.

Scheibel, M. E. and Scheibel, A. B. The response of reticular units to repetitive stimuli. Archives italiannes de Biologie, 103: 279-299, 1965.

Sherrington, C. S. The integrative action of the nervous system. (2nd Edition). New Haven, Connecticut, Yale University Press, 1947.

Siegel, J. M. and McGinty, D. J. Brainstem neurons without spontaneous unit discharge. Science, 193: 240-242, 1976.

Siegel, J. M. and McGinty, D. J. Pontine reticular formation neurons: Relationship of discharge to motor activity. Science, 196: 678-680, 1977.

Siegel, J. M., McGinty, D. J. and Breedlove, S.M. Sleep and waking activity of pontine giganto-cellular field neurons. Experimental Neurology, 56: 553-573, 1977.

Simon, R. P., Gershon, M. D. and Brooks, D. C. The role of the raphe nuclei in the regulation of ponto-geniculo-occipital wave activity. Brain Research, 58: 313-330, 1973.

Sprague, J. M. Interaction of cortex and superior colliculus in mediation of visually guided behavior in the cat. Science, 153: 1544-1547, 1966.

Villablanca, J. Behavioral and polygraphic study of "sleep" and "wakefulness" in chronic decerebrate cats. · Electroencephalography and Clinical Neurophysiology, 21: 562-577, 1966.

SLEEP AND EPILEPSY: AN EXPERIMENTAL STUDY

MARCOS VELASCO, FRANCISCO VELASCO
and FRANCISCO ESTRADA-VILLANUEVA

Division of Neurophysiology
Scientific Research Department
National Medical Center IMSS
México, D. F.

The relationship between sleep and epilepsy has been traditionally recognized: Hippocrates believed that epilepsy and sleep were equivalent states since both consisted in transient, reversible and periodic alterations of consciousness. Gowers (1901) described the frequency of nocturnal seizures, the time at which they occur and the possible triggering by dreams. Gibbs and Gibbs (1942) showed that sleep activates interictal epileptic EEG spikes and "sleep activation" has been utilized since as a diagnostic EEG procedure for detecting and localizing epileptogenic foci.

Numerous clinical studies have been done to determine the way sleep modifies the epileptic attacks but either sleep facilitation or inhibition on epilepsy has been reported depending on a number of factors as age and constitution of epileptic patients, nature of epileptic attacks, sensitivity to anticonvulsant regimes and phase of sleep considered. For example, Janz (1962) classified epileptic seizures in three types according to their behavior during the wakefulness-sleep cycle: 1. Nocturnal seizures present only during sleep (sleep facilitation), starting at any age, often cryptogenetic associated to psychomotor types which are sensitive to hydantoins. Patients with nocturnal seizures easily fall asleep and arouse with their major lucidity periods in the morning. 2. Diurnal seizures present only during wakefulness (sleep inhibition) starting from 14 to 25 years of age, often cryptogenetic associated to petit mal types. Patients with diurnal seizures hardly fall asleep and arouse with their major lucidity periods in the afternoon. 3. Diffuse seizures present either by day or by night (not modified by sleep) generally of a partial type

Copyright © 1979 by Academic Press, Inc.
All rights of reproduction in any form reserved.
ISBN 0-12-222340-3

and sensitive to barbiturates. In addition, different investigators have reported that the onset of
clinical seizures and the interictal EEG discharges
are facilitated during slow wave sleep (SWS) and
are inhibited during paradoxical sleep (PS). These
influences are particularly important in the case
of the temporal lobe discharges (Delange et al.,
1962a; Bancaud et al., 1965; Gastaut et al., 1965;
Passouant and Cadilhac, 1970c, and others). However, some epileptiform activities may be either
attenuated (continuous hypsarrhythmic discharges,
Gastaut et al., 1965) or not modified (period
bursts of subacute leukoencephalitis, Passouant
et al., 1970b) during both SWS and PS phases of
sleep. Furthermore, many EEG seizures are prominent during transitional phases of sleep
(Passouant and Cadilhac, 1970c) and arousal may
either facilitate petit mal (Tomka et al., 1971)
and myoclonic discharges (Gastaut and Tassinari,
1966a) or inhibit photo-myoclonic epileptic
episodes (Meir-Ewert and Broughton, 1967).

Experimental studies on sleep and epilepsy
have been highly confined to EEG phenomenology.
They have shown that SWS facilitates while PS
inhibits focal EEG after-discharges produced by
threshold convulsive activation of amygdala and
hippocampus in chronically implanted cats
(Passouant et al., 1957; Guerrero-Figueroa et al.,
1965; Hernandez-Peon et al., 1965; Ioselani et al.,
1974). In addition, arousal response blocks
various forms of focal interictal spikes in both
chronic (Guerrero-Figueroa et al., 1963) and
acute preparations (Arduini and Lairy-Bounes, 1952;
Lairy-Bounes et al., 1952; Whitlock et al., 1953;
Pinel and Chorover, 1975). Only one investigation
in cats has considered the effect of sleep on both
clinical and EEG symptoms of epilepsy (Courtois,
1972).

In the course of our studies on alumina cream
induced focal motor epilepsy in cats (Velasco
et al., 1973a, b, 1976), it has been noticed that
one type of cortical paroxysmal EEG spikes from
epileptogenic focus (spikes) was consistently
accompanied by flexor tonic contractions of the
contralateral facial, neck and forelimb muscles
(convulsions) when animals were awake, while spikes
appear in absence of convulsions when animals were

asleep. This fact and other methodological advan-
tages of this model of experimental epilepsy has
motivated a systematic study on the effect of
wakefulness-sleep states on electrophysiological
and clinical manifestations of epilepsy (Velasco,
et al., 1977a, b, c, d, e).

A reliable method of experimental epilepsy

Single microinjections of 0.03 - 0.04 ml of
alumina cream into the sensory motor cortex of the
cat (4 mm lateral to the midline, 1 mm anterior to
the cruciate sulcus and 4 mm in depth) invariably
produce focal motor seizures. This form of experimental epilepsy seems suitable to study the anatomical and physiological mechanisms of focal epilepsy in the cat since animals show: 1) Small
epileptogenic lesions with a total area of 11.5 mm^2
and a length of 3.0 mm, confined to the anterior
sigmoid cortex and white matter subjacent to anterior sigmoid, anterior limbic and orbitofrontal
cortices (figure 1). 2) Clinical convulsions develop 34.5 $\pm$ days and last to 50.5 $\pm$ 5 days after
alumina cream injection. The clinical course is
therefore divided in 3 consecutive, sharply de-
lineated stages: Latent, convulsive and remission
stages. EEG spike density at the focus (number/
10 min) significantly increases before, reaches
maximum during and significantly decreases after
the convulsive stage (figure 2). 3) During the
convulsive stage solely focal (or focally initiated)
seizures are present and may be classified in 3
types according to their EEG patterns as follows:
Type A consisting in incremental, rhythmical 4/sec
spikes correlates to bilateral (predominantly
contralateral) rhythmic convulsions of face, neck
and forelimb muscles, resembles human "petit mal
like" seizures originating from parasagittal pre-
frontal and orbitofrontal regions (Penfield and
Jasper, 1954). Type B consisting in isolated
spikes correlates to isolated contralateral convulsions of same muscle groups, resembles human
"epilepsia partialis continua" originating from
the motor cortex (Koshewnikov, 1895). Type C
consisting in prolonged repetitive spikes correlates to repetitive convulsions of same muscle
groups, resembles human "adversive" seizures originating from intermediate frontal zone (Penfield
and Jasper, 1954).

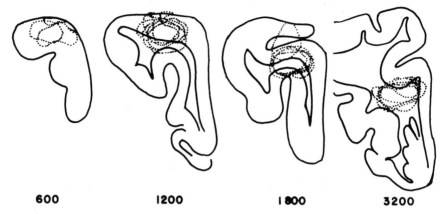

600   **1200**   **1800**   **3200**

Fig. 1 Diagrams of coronal sections taken
at 600, 1200, 1800 and 3200 microns from the tip of
the frontal lobe showing the site and extent of
alumina cream lesions in 8 cats (superimposed
dotted lines). (After Velasco et al., 1977a).

During latent and remission stages types a
and b similar to A and B discharges are present
only when animals are asleep and are not accompanied by convulsions. Types a and b are immediately
preceded by "spike spindles" and are followed by
"slow spindles". EEG and behavior of these animals
are normal in early latent and late remission
stages with no evidence of self sustained EEG focus
or residual neurological deficits (figure 3).

Anatomical alterations at the epileptogenic focus

If one compares the alumina cream epileptogenic lesions and adjacent cortical tissue of cats
sacrificed during latent, convulsive and remission
stages the following analogies and differences may
be found: On one hand, lesions show similar size
and histopathological elements during different
stages: a central deposit of alumina cream with
macrophages, absence of fibrotic capsule at the
edge and few or no inflammatory cells in the perilesional cortical tissue (figure 4). On the other
hand, the cortical tissue adjacent to lesions show
differential changes according to stage: During
the convulsive stage, the adjacent cerebral cortex
shows at the light microscopy a reduction of

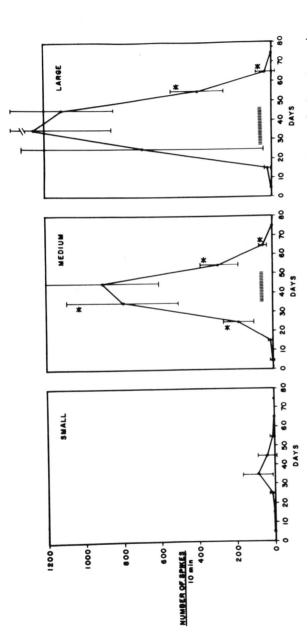

Fig. 2. Continuous lines: spike density (spikes/10 min) at epileptogenic focus (anterior sigmoid gyrus) determined every 10 days, for
a total period of 80 days in groups of cats after injection of small
(0.01 ml), medium (0.03 ml) and large (0.10 ml) quantities of alumina
cream. Mean ± standard error of the mean. Asterisk: significant
changes (p ≤ 0.01). Dashed area: occurrence of clinical convulsions.
(After Velasco et al., 1973a).

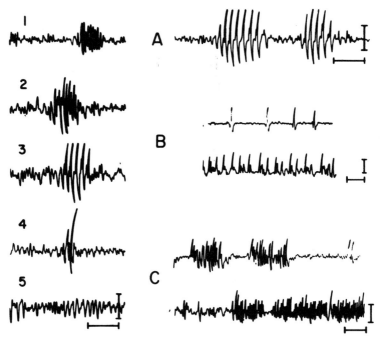

Fig. 3. Types of spikes at the epileptogenic focus (anterior sigmoid gyrus) of cat
P21 during latent, convulsive and remission
stages. Right: awake records taken during
convulsive stage showing type A, B and C EEG
spikes. Left: asleep records taken during
latent (1-3) and remission stages (4-5) showing type a (3) and type b spikes (4), normal
spindles (1), spiky spindles (2) and slow
spindles. (After Velasco et al., 1977a).

overall thickness and cellularity which is significantly more important on non-pyramidal neurons
located at layers II and IV than on the pyramidal
ones located at layer V (figure 5). At the
electron microscopy pyramidal cells show evidence
of a slow progressive degeneration (increase density of cytoplasmic matrix, disorganization of
intraterminal elements, dilation of vesicles and
distortion of mitochondria). In addition, there is
an increase number of glial processes not only
surrounding the blood vessels but also intermingled

with neuropil elements (figures 6 and 7). During the latent stage these changes are only incipient while during the remission stage there is a total neuronal depopulation at the perilesional cortical tissue.

Cerebral lesions produced by silicon with similar location and extent of those produced by alumina cream are followed by neither clinical nor EEG signs of epilepsy. Silicon lesions of cats sacrificed 40 days after lesion produce an intense chronic inflammatory reactions with fibrotic capsule, vascular proliferation and interstitial edema of the perilesional nervous tissue. The adjacent cortex shows massive destruction of all pyramidal and non-pyramidal elements (figures 4S and 5S).

These results indicate that occurrence of EEG and clinical seizures in this model of epilepsy is independent on the scar formation or inflammatory alterations of the cortical tissue. In addition, they suggest that absence of EEG and clinical seizures after silicon lesions and during the remission stage of alumina cream lesions is due to either total damage or total depopulation of they pyramidal and non-pyramidal elements of the adjacent cortical tissue. On the contrary, the precise mechanism by which alumina cream lesions produce EEG and clinical seizures remains unknown. However, these data suggest that there is a number of anatomical factors produced by the alumina cream which may participate in the physiopathology of the epileptic focus. For example, disruption of intracortical regulatory circuitry, alterations in excitable properties of the synaptic membrane of the pyramidal neurons and changes in the local electro-lytic environment due to glial proliferation (Velasco et al., 1973a, b, 1976, 1977f).

Wakefulness-sleep modulation of epileptic activity

In addition to the anatomical alterations within the epileptogenic focus, other extrafocal physiological factors have to be considered in the physiopathogenesis of EEG and clinical paroxysms as those depending on the wakefulness-sleep state of the animals. However, while the focal anatomic-al factors affect EEG and clinical paroxysms in a parallel way (both are low during latent, both

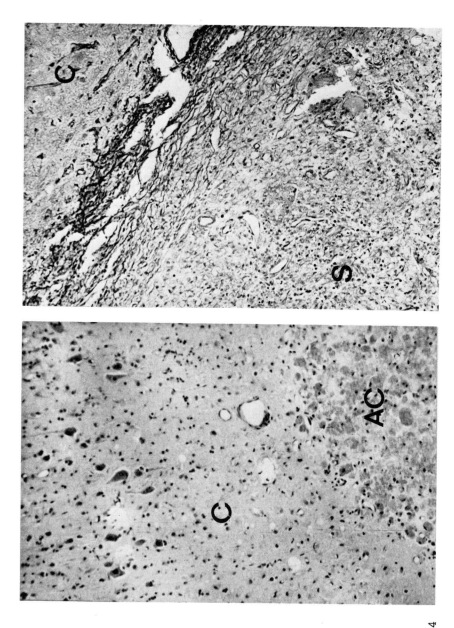

Fig. 4

Fig. 4. Light microscopic view of the edge of alumina cream (AC) and silicon (S) lesions. AC lesion shows a central deposit with AC-loaded macrophages, absence of fibrotic capsule at the edge and only scarce inflammatory nuclear cells in the perilesional cortical tissue (C). Silicon lesions show a central necrotic area with numerous blood vessels and inflammatory cells and scattered giant cells. At the edge, there is a conspicuous thick fibrotic capsule. The perilesional cortical tissue shows interstitial edema and numerous mononuclear cells. AC lesion stained with hematoxyline-eosine and silicon lesions with Gomory's technique x 400. (After Velasco et al., 1973b).

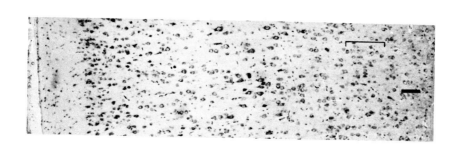

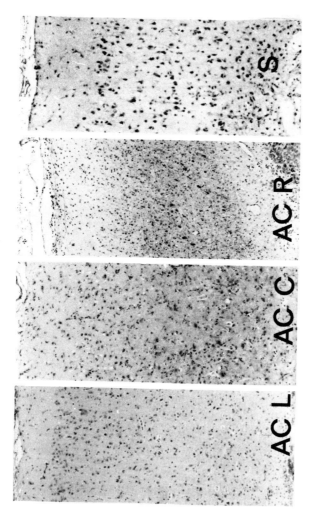

Fig. 5. Light microscopic view of the cortical tissue adjacent to alumina cream lesions showing comparatively its thickness and cellularity in five different animals. Left: cerebral cortex of those with alumina cream lesions sacrificed during latent (ACL), convulsive (ACC) and remission stages (ACR) and an animal with silicon lesion (S) sacrificed 40 days after operation. Right: cerebral cortex of an intact animal (I) also sacrificed 40 days after operation. Hematoxyline-eosine stains. Calibration: 200 microns. (After Velasco et al., 1973b).

82

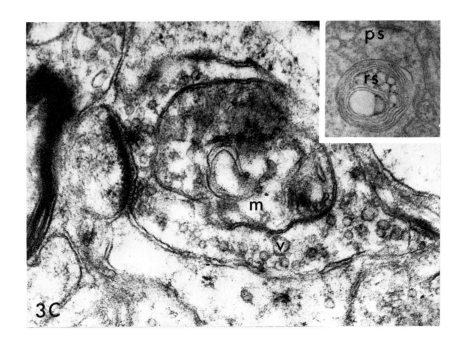

Fig. 6. Electron microscopic detail of the cortical elements adjacent to alumina cream lesion of a brain examined during the convulsive stage showing degenerative changes in a synaptic terminal (S) with a marked distorted mitochondrion (m). Arrow = intersynaptic space. Lead citrate and uranyl acetate (x 35,000). (After Velasco et al., 1976).

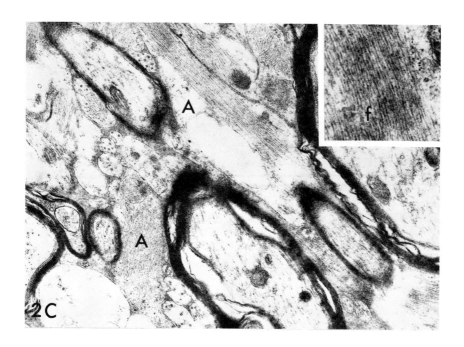

Fig. 7. Electron microscopic detail of the cortical elements adjacent to alumina cream lesion of a brain examined during the convulsive stage showing numerous astrocytic processes (G) in the neuropil. Inset: arrow shows glial filaments within an astrocytic process. Lead citrate and uranyl acetate (x 17,500, inset x 50,000). (After Velasco et al., 1976).

increase during convulsive and both decrease during
remission stages) the wakefulness-sleep physiological factors affect EEG and clinical paroxysms
in a different way, depending upon the type of
epileptic attack and the wakefulness-sleep state.
For example, in the case of type B epilepsy, wakefulness (W) and arousal (AR) decrease EEG spikes
and increase EMG convulsions, slow wave sleep (SWS)
increases spikes and decreases convulsions and
paradoxical sleep (PS) decreases both spikes
and convulsions. (figures 8 and 9). Since the

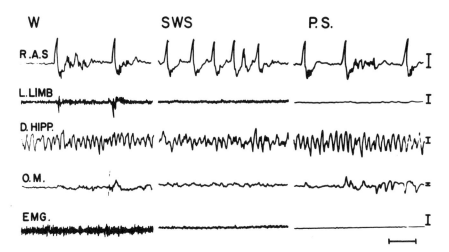

Fig. 8. EEG spikes from epileptic focus (RAS)
and muscle clonic contractions from left limb (L.
LIMB) during different wakefulness-sleep states:
wakefulness (W), slow wave sleep (SWS) and paradoxical sleep (PS) in the same cat. Correlation
between individual spikes and convulsions is equal
to one during W and is equal to zero (or near zero)
during SWS and PS. Other electrophysiological parameters show a clear cut differentiation between
wakefulness-sleep states, i.e., electrical activity
of dorsal hippocampus (D. HIPP), ocular movements
(OM) and tone of neck muscles (EMG). (After
Velasco et al., 1977a).

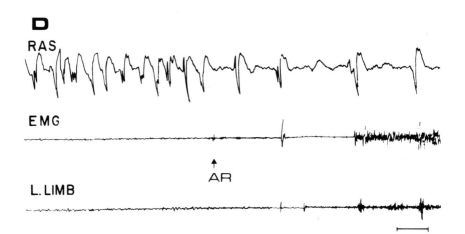

Fig. 9. Sequential changes in type B spikes from right epileptic focus (RAS), clinical convulsions from left forelimb (L. Limb) and tone of neck muscles (EMG) during arousal (AR): 1. Arousal stimulus presentation, 2. Decrease number of type B spikes immediately after arousal, 3. Increases amplitude of muscle contractions 2-5 sec. after arousal, and 4. Further increase amplitude of muscle contractions and increase tonus of neck muscles 5-10 sec. after arousal. Calibration: 1 sec. (After Velasco et al., 1977a).

amplitude, duration and interval variance of EEG spikes are not modified while animals shift through these different wakefulness-sleep states, it can be visualized that occurrence of clinical convulsions does not depend on changes detected by the conventional EEG. Therefore, there was the possibility that either EEG spikes are not reliable indicators of the initiation of cortical epileptic impulses or the propagation of epileptic impulses may be modulated at the level of the spinal cord during different wakefulness-sleep states.

On the assumption that muscular clonic contractions are due to high frequency hypersynchronic impulses time locked to the EEG spike originated in the cerebral cortex and transmitted to the

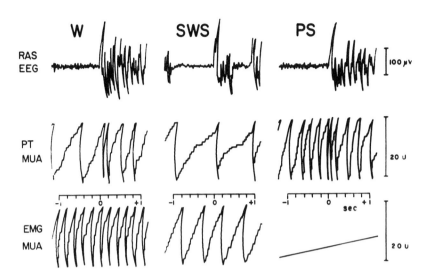

Fig. 10. Conventional EEG traces from epileptic focus (RAS EEG) and integrated multiple unit activities from ipsilateral pyramidal tract (PTMUA) and neck muscles (EMGMUA) from one cat during W, SWS and PS. Tonic MUA was defined as the total number of pyramidal or muscular active units per minute. Phasic MUA was defined as transient increments in number of pyramidal units time locked to the onset of cortical EEG spike (time 0). Increments in number of pyramidal units were determined every 200 milliseconds from 1 sec. before (-1) to 1 sec. after (+1) zero. The oblique straight line in EMGMUA during PS indicate the baseline of the integrator. (After Velasco et al., 1977b).

muscles through a cortico spinal pyramidal pathway (Adrian and Moruzzi, 1939), electrodes were implanted in a group of cats for recording multiple unit activity, at the pyramidal tract (PTMUA) for

detecting cortically originated epileptic impulses
and at the posterior cervical muscles (EMGMUA) for
evaluation of the excitability in alpha motoneurons enervating extensor and flexor muscles
during wakefulness and sleep (Morrison and Pompeiano, 1965).

    It was found that W and AR increase both PT
and EMG MUAs, SWS decreases both PT and EMGMUAs
and PS increases PT but decreases EMGMUA (figures
10 and 11). Therefore, it can be concluded that
presence of clinical convulsions during W is due
to a facilitation of the cortical initiation and
spinal propagation of epileptic impulses, absence of
clinical convulstions during SWS is due to inhibition of both while during PS is due to facilitation of cortical initiation and inhibition of
spinal propagation of epileptic impulses.

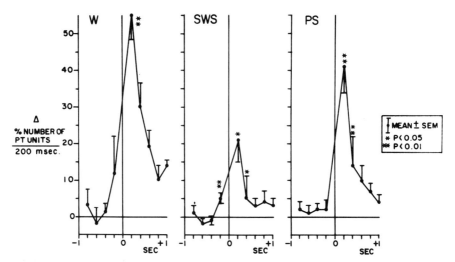

    Fig. 11. Phasic changes in PTMUA from the
group of cats during wakefulness-sleep states
considered separately. Consecutive increments in
per cent number of PT units/200 msec. determined
from 1 sec. before (-1) to 1 sec. after (+1) the
onset of cortical EEG spike (0). (After Velasco
et al., 1977b).

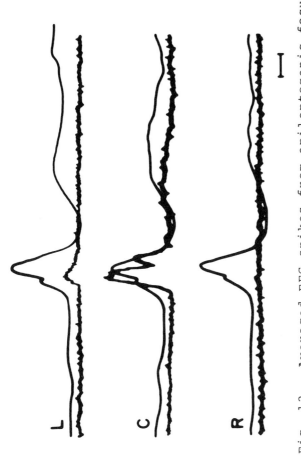

Fig. 12. Averaged EEG spikes from epiloptogenic focus and integrated multiple unit activity from the pyramidal tract from one cat during latent, convulsive and remission stages. Calibration: 100 msec. (After Velasco et al., 1977d).

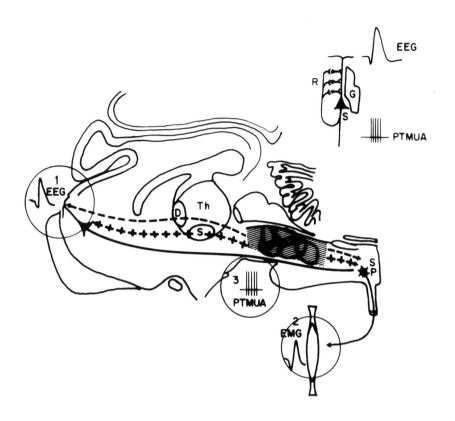

Figure 13

Fig. 13 Wakefulness-sleep mechanisms modulating focal motor epilepsy.

Top right: Diagram of cellular organization of motor cortex illustrating the main anatomical changes in neural tissue adjacent to epileptogenic lesions. S = slow degenerative changes in soma of pyramidal cells at the V cortical layer. R = significant loss of non pyramidal cells at the II and IV cortical layers. G = proliferation of microglial elements (fibrotic astrocytes). These anatomical changes correlate with two possible different electrophysiological events: EEG spikes and PTMUA phasic discharges.

Bottom left: Diagram of parasagittal view of cats brain illustrating the possible neurophysiological mechanisms by which wakefulness-sleep states regulate the initiation and propagation of epileptic impulses. 1) Cortical initiation of epileptic impulses time locked to the EEG spike. 2) Pyramidal propagation of cortical epileptic impulses. 3) Effect of epileptic impulses on spinal motoneuron (SP) reflected as a muscular EMG contraction.

RF = Brain stem reticular nuclei mediating cortical and spinal regulatory influences during W, AR, SWS and PS.

Ascending interrupted lines = Regulation of apical dendritic cortical synapses through the diffuse thalamic projection system (D).

Ascending crossed lines = Regulation of basal dendritic cortical synapses through the specific thalamic projection system (S).

Descending interrupted lines = Regulation of the spinal motoneuron through inhibitory reticulo spinal pathways.

Descending crossed lines = Regulation of the spinal motoneuron through excitatory reticulo spinal pathways.

COMMENT

Eventhough present results are confined to only one form of experimental epilepsy, they allow to formulate a hypothesis on basic mechanisms by which wakefulness-sleep states modulate other forms of experimental and clinical epilepsies. In order to fit all these experimental facts in a congruent scheme, it is necessary to assume that EEG spikes and action potentials of PT neurons are two related but independent events. In fact, dissociation between these two events has been previously reported in a number of epileptiform potentials (Adrian and Moruzzi, 1939; Whitlock et al., 1953; Ajmone-Marsan, 1969, and others). In present experiments EEG spikes and PT action potentials are also dissociated during SWS in latent, convulsive and remission stages and during arousal in the convulsive stage (figure 12). Furthermore, diazepam -an anticonvulsant utilized in the control of clinical seizures- like SWS increases EEG spikes and reduces PT action potentials (Velasco et al., 1977c). Electrophysiologically, EEG spikes seem to be related to activation of the apical dendrites of PT neurons by the diffuse thalamic projection nuclei regulating the local excitatory cortical state, while PT action potentials seem to be related to activation of the basal dendrites of PT neurons by the specific thalamic projection nuclei determining the propagated cortico spinal impulses (c.f. Creutzfeld, 1974).

The relationship of EEG spikes-EMG convulsions is clear in this model of experimental epilepsy since EMG convulsions occur only in presence of EEG spikes. Therefore it can be postulated that EEG spikes increase probability for occurrence of EMG convulsions. Other factors, however, have to be considered in the determination of EMG convulsions as the presence of the above mentioned PT cortico spinal impulses and the local excitatory state of the spinal motoneurons which in the case of wakefulness-sleep states depends upon descending reticulo spinal inhibition-excitation balance (Magoun, 1958).

Figure 13 summarizes the proposal of the basic mechanisms of wakefulness-sleep modulation of focal motor seizures: Top right: anatomical alterations at the epileptogenic focus produce a continuous generation of local EEG spikes and propagated PT impulses. Bottom left: PT impulses are propagated to muscles through PT cortico spinal tract (1-2-3). Wakefulness reduces EEG spikes through the diffuse thalamic projection system (D) while increases PT impulses through the specific thalamic projection system (S) and spinal cord excitability through the facilitatory reticulo spinal system (RF+). As a consequence, wakefulness decreases probability for EMG convulsions to occur but at the same time facilitates the mechanisms for EMG convulsions. Slow wave sleep increases EEG spikes through D while decreases PT impulses through S and spinal cord excitability through the inhibitory reticulo spinal system (RF-). As a consequence, slow wave sleep increases probability for EMG convulsions to occur but at the same time inhibits the mechanism for EMG convulsions. Parodoxical sleep decreases EEG spikes through D, PT impulses through S and spinal cord excitability through RF-. As a consequence, paradoxical sleep decreases probability and inhibits the mechanism of EMG convulsions.

REFERENCES

Adrian, E. D. and Moruzzi, G. Impulses in the pyramidal tract. <u>Journal</u> <u>of</u> <u>Physiology</u>, <u>London</u>, <u>97</u>: 153-199, 1939.

Ajmone-Marsan, C. Acute effects of topical epileptogenic agents. In Jasper, H. H. and Ward, A. A. Jr. and Pope, A. (Eds.) <u>Basic</u> <u>Mechanisms</u> <u>of</u> <u>the</u> <u>Epilepsies</u>. Boston: Little Brown, 1969, pp. 299-319.

Arduini, A. et Lairy-Bounes, G. C. Action de la stimulation electrique de la formation reticulaire du bulbe et des stimulations sensorielles sur les ondes strychniques corticales chez le chat "encephale isole". <u>Electroencephalography</u> <u>and</u> <u>Clinical</u> <u>Neurophysiology</u>, <u>4</u>: 503-512, 1952.

Bancaud, J., Talairach, J., Bordas-Ferrer, M., Auber, J. L. et Marchand, H. Les acces epileptiques au cours du sommeil de nuit. In: Le Sommeil de Nuit Normal et Pathologique: Etudes electroencephalographiques. Paris: Masson, 1965, pp. 255-274.

Courtois, A. Motor phenomenology of cobalt experimental epileptic focus in the motor cortex of the cat during various stages of vigilance. Electroencephalography and Clinical Neurophysiology, 32: 259-267, 1972.

Creutzfeld, O. and Houchin, J. Neuronal bases of EEG-waves. In Remond, A. (Ed.) Handbook of Electroencephalography and Clinical Neurophysiology, Volume 2, Part C, pp. 5-55, 1974.

Delange, M., Castan, P., Cadilhac, J. et Passouant, P. Les divers stades du sommeil chez le nouveau-nee et le nourrison. Revue Neurologie (Paris) 107: 271-276, 1962.

Gastaut, H. et Tassinari, C. A. Triggering mechanism in epilepsy: the electroclinical point of view. Epilepsia (Amsterdam) 7: 85-138, 1966.

Gastaut, H., Batini, C., Broughton, R., Fressy, J. et Tassinari, C. A. Etudes electroencephalographiques des phenomenes non epileptiques au cours du sommeil. In: Le Sommeil de Nuit Normal et Pathologique: Etudes electroencephalographiques. Paris: Masson, 1965, pp. 215-238.

Gibbs, F. A. and Gibbs, E. L. Atlas of Electroencephalography. Cambridge: Addison-Wesley, 1942.

Gowers, W. Epilepsy and other chronic convulsive diseases. London: Churchill, 1901, Vol I.

Guerrero-Figueroa, R., Barros, A. and De Balbian-V ester, F. Some inhibitory effects of attentive factors on experimental epilepsy. Epilepsia (Amsterdam, 4: 225-240, 1963.

Guerrero-Figueroa, R., Lester, B. and Heath, R. Changes of hippocampal epileptiform activity during wakefulness and sleep. Acta Neurologica Latino Americana, 11: 330-337, 1965.

Hernandez-Peon, R. and Guerrero-Figueroa, R. Modification of local amygdaloid evoked responses during wakefulness and sleep. Acta Neurologica Latino Americana, 11: 224-232, 1965.

Ioselani, T. K., Nanovashvili, Z. I. and Khizanishvili, N. A. Changes in seizure activity thresholds of the cat brain in various stages of sleep and wakefulness. Neurophysiologiya, 6: 577-584, 1974.

Janz, D. The Grand-Mal epilepsies and the sleeping-waking cycle. Epilepsia (Amsterdam), 3: 69-109, 1962.

Koshewnikov, E. Eine besondere form von corticales epilepsy. Neurol. Zbl., 14: 47-48, 1895.

Lairy-Bounes, C. G., Parma, M. et Zanchetti, A. Modificationspendant la reaction d'arret de Berger de l'activite convulsive produite par l'application locale de strychnine sur le cortex du lapin. Electroencephalography and Clinical Neurophysiology, 4: 495-502, 1952.

Magoun, H. W. The Waking Brain. Springfield, Ill: Charles Thomas, 1958, pp. 15-23.

Meier-Ewert, K. and Broughton, R. Photomyo-clonic response of epileptic and non-epileptic subjects during wakefulness, sleep, and arousal. Electroencephalography and Clinical Neurophysiology, 23: 142-151, 1967.

Morrison, A. R. and Pompeiano, O. An analyses of the supraspinal influences acting on motoneurons during sleep in the unrestrained cat. Responses on the alpha motoneurons to direct electrical stimulation during sleep. Archives Italiannes de Biologie, 103: 497-516, 1965.

Passouant, P. et Cadilhac, J. Decharges epi-leptiques et sommeil Epilepsie, Modern Problems in Pharmaco-psychiatry, 4: 87-104, 1970.

Passouant, P., Passouant-Fontaine, Th. et Cadilhac, J. Sommeil et epilepsie experimentale hippocampique. Role de l'eveil dans la production des decharges hippocampiques. Comptes Rendus des Seances de la Societe de Biologie (Paris), 151: 2166-2169, 1957.

Penfield, W. and Jasper, H. H. Epilepsy and the functional anatomy of the human brain. Boston: Little Brown, 1954, pp. 606-607 and 827.

Pinel, J. P. J. and Chorover, S. L. Inhibition by arousal of epilepsy induced by chlorambucil in rats. Nature (London), 236: 232-234, 1975.

Tomka, I., Passouant, P. and Baldy-Moulinier, M. REM and petit-mal epilepsy. 1st International Congress of the Association for the Psychophysiological Study of Sleep, Bruges, Belgium, 1971.

Velasco, M., Velasco, F., Estrada-Villanueva, F. and Olvera, A. Alumina cream-induced focal motor epilepsy in cats. 1. Lesion size and temporal course. Epilepsia (Amsterdam), 14: 3-14, 1973a.

Velasco, M., Velasco, F., Lozoya, X., Feria, A. and Gonzalez-Licea, A. Alumina cream-induced focal motor epilepsy in cats. 2. Thickness and cellularity of cerebral cortex adjacent to epileptogenic lesions. Epilepsia (Amsterdam), 14: 15-27, 1973b.

Velasco, M., Velasco, F. and Feria-Velasco, A. Alumina cream-induced focal motor epilepsy in cats. 3. Ultrastructure of the epileptogenic focus. Archivos de Investigacion Medica (Mexico), 7: 157-170, 1976.

Velasco, M., Velasco, F., Cepeda, C., Almanza, X. and Estrada-Villanueva, F. Alumina cream-induced focal motor epilepsy in cats. I. Wakefulness-sleep modulation of cortical paroxysmal EEG spikes. Electroencephalography and Clinical Neurophysiology, 43: 59-66, 1977a.

Velasco, M., Velasco, F., Cepeda, C. and Estrada-Villanueva, F. Alumina cream-induced focal motor epilepsy in cats. II. Wakefulness-sleep modulation of pyramidal tract multiple unit activity. Electroencephalography and Clinical Neurophysiology, 43: 67-73, 1977b.

Velasco, M., Velasco, F., Cepeda, C. and De Anda, J. A.: Effect of diazepam on pyramidal tract and electromyographic multiple unit activities of cats with chronic epileptogenic foci. Neuropharmamacology, 16: 299-301, 1977c.

Velasco, M., Velasco, F., Cepeda, C. and Estrada-Villanueva, F. Alumina cream-induced focal motory epilepsy in cats. III. Development of EEG spikes and pyramidal tract multiple unit activity. Electroencephalography and Clinical Neurophysiology, (submitted for publication), 1977d.

Velasco, M., Velasco, F., Cepeda, C. and Estrada-Villanueva, F. Alumina cream-induced focal motor epilepsy in cats. IV. Pyramidal and extrapyramidal propagation of epileptic impulses. Electroencephalography and Clinical Neurophysiology, (submitted for publication), 1977e.

Velasco, M., Velasco, F. and Feria-Velasco, A. Alumina cream-induced focal motor epilepsy in cats. 4. Cellularity of different layers of cerebral cortex adjacent to epileptogenic focus. Epilepsia (New York), (submitted for publication), 1977f.

Whitlock, D. G., Arduini, A. and Moruzzi, G. Microelectrode analyses of pyramidal system during transition from sleep to wakefulness. Journal of Neurophysiology, 16: 414-429, 1953.

PROTEIN MOLECULES AND THE REGULATION OF REM SLEEP: POSSIBLE IMPLICATIONS FOR FUNCTION

RENE DRUCKER-COLIN

Departamento de Biología Experimental
Instituto de Biología
Universidad Nacional Autónoma de México
México, D. F.

For quite some time now, studies which have attempted to investigate about the neurochemical control or regulation of sleep have mostly focused on the monoamines. As we all know, in recent years peptides and even protein molecules have captured the attention of various fields of neuroscience. Nevertheless, aside from the numerous reports on sleep related release of hormones, which parenthetically have so far contributed little to knowledge about the neurohumoral control of sleep, sleep research has paid relatively little attention to peptides and protein molecules as potential factors involved in the regulation of sleep.

In this chapter I will attempt to convince the reader about the idea that there may be other molecules, beside the biogenic amines, which may play a crucial role in the processes which lead to REM sleep, and that they may be worthwhile pursuing. Approximately ten years ago Oswald (1969) suggested that the rebound of REM sleep which occurrs following the withdrawal of chronic drug adminis- tration, was the result of a repair process, which involved an increase in the intensity of brain synthetic activity. This concept has recently been extended (Adam and Oswald, 1977) by suggesting, that rest and sleep in a variety of species, represents a period of peak anabolic functions. Evidence has been slowly accumulating, supporting Oswald's suggestion.

First, Brodskii et al (1974) have shown that REM sleep, as opposed to slow wave sleep is accom- panied by an increase of brain protein synthesis, whereas Voronka et al (1971) while studying the content of protein in individual neurons and neuro- glia, reported that sleep was accompanied by an

Copyright © 1979 by Academic Press, Inc.
All rights of reproduction in any form reserved.
ISBN 0-12-222340-3

increase in proteins, and REM sleep deprivation by
a decrease. More recently we have shown that
levels of proteins in push-pull perfusates obtained
from the midbrain reticular formation during the
sleep-wake cycle, vary in a cyclic manner, and that
the peaks of protein levels occurr at times when
REM sleep occupies the greatest portion of time
(Drucker-Colin et al, 1975; Drucker-Colin and
Spanis, 1976). Moreover when sleep is disturbed by
basal forebrain lesions (McGinty and Sterman, 1968),
the cyclic variations in proteins disappear (Drucker-
Colin and Gutierrez, 1976).

A second line of evidence comes from several
reports which have shown that a single administration of protein synthesis inhibitors, have a specific REM sleep inhibitory effect in mice (Pegram
et al, 1973), rats (Rojas-Ramirez et al, 1977;
Kitahama and Valatx, 1975) and cats (Petitjean et
al, 1975; Drucker-Colín et al, 1978). One report
even showed a sort of rebound effect, since REM
sleep was increased for several days following administration of cycloheximide (Stern et al, 1972).
It is interesting, that at least three of these
reports, which have analyzed the causes for the
reduction of REM sleep, have shown that it comes
through a decrease in the frequency of REM periods
and not through the duration of individual periods.
These observations provide support for the notion
that proteins or their synthesis participate in
the triggering of REM sleep, rather than on its
maintenance (though this may be argued; see below).
This is further supported by the fact that REM
sleep rebound following either sleep deprivation
(Fig. 1) or following withdrawal from chronic
amphetamine administration (Fig. 2) is completely
blocked by chloramphenicol (Drucker-Colin and
Benitez, 1977).

Should proteins be involved in the mechanisms
which trigger REM sleep, one might ask how this
comes about. We have in our laboratory performed
a few experiments attempting to provide answers to
this question. It is well known that REM sleep is
accompanied by a variety of phasic events such as
PGO waves, myoclonic jerks, bursts of eye movements
and bursts of high frequency unit activity. This
allows division of REM sleep into two clearly distinct
and continuously oscillating periods (Fig. 3),
referred to as phasic REM (REM_p) and tonic REM (REM_t).

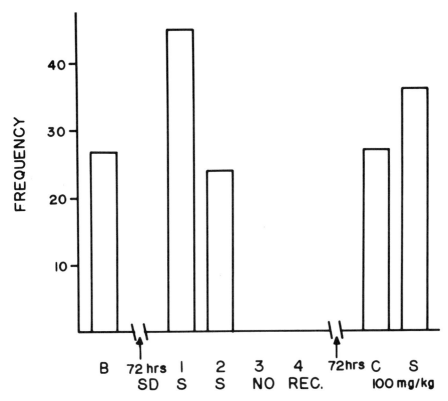

Fig. 1.   Histogram showing the frequency of
REM periods before and after 72 hours of sleep
deprivation (SD), in control and chloramphenicol
(C) treated cats. Saline (S)

In this latter phase, the decrease and/or absence
of phasic events is quite notable. We have recently
calculated that approximately 40% of REM sleep is
occupied by REM_p (Fig. 4). However when protein
synthesis inhibitors are administered the amount of
REM_p diminishes very significantly (Fig. 4).   A
clear example of this can be seen in Figure 5.
Here, two REM sleep polygraphic samples, with (A)
or without (B) protein synthesis inhibitors are
shown.   The decrease in phasic events, i.e. PGO
and eye movement density and multiple unit activity

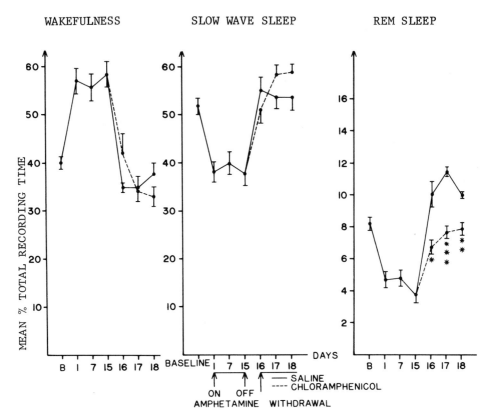

Fig. 2 Graph showing the percent of time spent in each
phase of the sleep-wake cycle.   The 12 animals in this
experiment following a baseline recording were injected
daily with 10 mg/kg of amphetamine.   Sleep recordings were
done only on days 1, 7, and 15. At this point the rats
were divided into two groups of 6.   One group received
daily injections of saline, the other of chloramphenicol
(100 mg. kg) and sleep recorded on days 16,17,18.   Note
decrease of sleep by amphetamine, rebound in SWS, but
absence of REM rebound in the chloramphenicol treated rats.

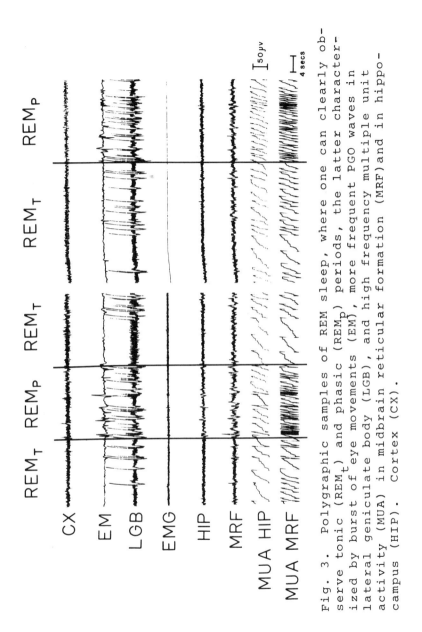

Fig. 3. Polygraphic samples of REM sleep, where one can clearly observe tonic (REM$_t$) and phasic (REM$_p$) periods, the latter characterized by burst of eye movements (EM), more frequent PGO waves in lateral geniculate body (LGB), and high frequency multiple unit activity (MUA) in midbrain reticular formation (MRF) and in hippocampus (HIP). Cortex (CX).

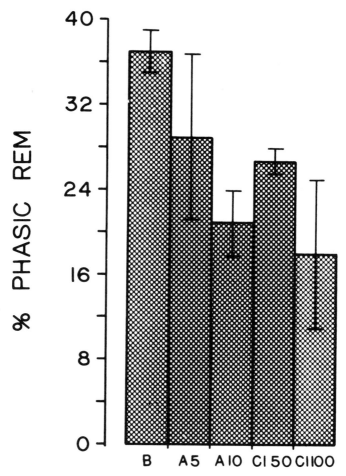

Fig. 4. Histogram showing that protein synthesis inhibitors decrease phasic REM sleep time. Baseline (B), Anisomycin 5 mg/kg (A5) Anisomycin 10 mg/kg (A10), chloramphenicol 50 mg/kg (CL50), chloramphenicol 100 mg/kg (CL100).

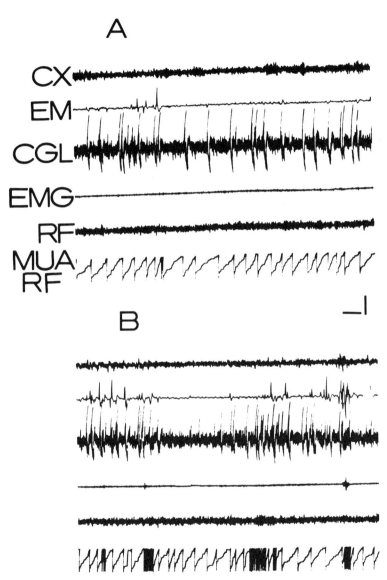

Fig. 5. Polygraphic REM sleep samples with (A) or without (B) cloramphenicol. Note diminished phasic activities in A.

(MUA) is noteworthy. It should additionally be pointed out that protein synthesis inhibitors retard the appearance of the first REM sleep period by several hours. During this time lag several abortive REM's occur. To put it in the vernacular, it looks as if cats have a difficultime entering into REM sleep. Moreover, when the first REM sleep finally shows up, it is usually very short and with an almost total absence of phasic events. In time, however, as decay of peak drug effects are initiated, the percent of phasic events begins to increase 'til they reach normality as phasic events begin to normalize, so do REM sleep durations. Preliminary analysis of our data indicates that of least about 20% REM_p should be present for REM sleep duration to be normal.

It was mentioned earlier that mean REM duration was unaffected by protein synthesis inhibitors. The fact that the first few REM's with important decreases of phasic events are of very short duration, seems to oppose this concept. This may be reconciled by suggesting that phasic events trigger REM, and that duration is dependent on them, up to a certain point. Thus protein synthesis inhibitors affect duration only to the extent that they affect the phasic elements of REM sleep.

With this in mind, it is conceivable that protein molecules, normally act as a "gate" or "signal" to let forth a chain of events which brings about what we have come to recognize as REM sleep. This chain of events could be the appearance of type II PGO waves, which have been suggested to drive the bursts of eye movements (Magherini et al, 1971), the increased frequency of unit activities which occurr a few seconds prior to REM sleep (Hobson et al, 1974), and the release of cholinergic and/or aminergic neurotransmitters (Jouvet, 1972). Visualized in this way, REM sleep would not depend on the release of one neurotransmitter from one specific brain structure, but would rather depend on a variety of events. The fact that there is equivocal data about the role of monoamines in sleep, may merely reflect the fact that only one of the elements involved in its regulation is studied in time and space.

We feel that further knowledge about the biochemical regulation of sleep, will not come about by belaboring on the theme of monoamines, but rather on how they interact with protein molecules, since it is evident that such molecules play an important role in sleep.

The possibility that proteins play a role in sleep, and in particular in REM sleep, is certainly an attractive one. It not only allows one to speculate, as we have, about their role in triggering REM sleep, or provide new possibilities for studying the biochemical regulation óf sleep, i.e. interaction with neurotransmitters, but also provides a means for speculating about the function of REM sleep.

Quite some time ago, Roffwarg et al (1966) suggested a role for REM sleep in development. This suggestion was partly based on the fact that newborn babies or animals, spend the greatest part of their days in REM sleep. This does not occur in guinea pigs, whose brain is fully matured at birth (Jouvet-Mounier et al, 1970). It is also weĺl known that brain protein synthesis is highest on the first few days after birth (Johnson and Lutgges, 1966). Although there is no data allowing to determine whether newborn animals sleep more because there is more protein synthesis or viceversa, we do know that they occurr concomittantly (Drucker-Colin, 1975). Therefore during the periods of accelerated brain development (neonatal period) REM sleep could subserve the function of aiding such development as suggested by Roffwarg. It remains to be seen whether REM sleep deprivation thwarts growth. Such an experiment, though fraught with difficulties, is badly needed, and would provide invaluable information.

As the organism grows, both REM sleep and protein synthesis rate decrease. However, as mentioned previously, protein synthesis or protein availability in brain is greater during REM sleep. Therefore, now in a fully developed brain, protein availability during REM sleep, may have acquired a new function. This function, maybe not akin to growth, would be, however, more oriented to the brain. The role of proteins in REM sleep could be to aid memory consolidation (Bloch, 1977; Bloch and Fishbein, 1976; Fishbein and Gutwein, 1977) and to guard the integrity of the neural circuitry which subserves this function.

Viewed in this way, REM sleep comes to acquire a daily (nightly) function of utmost importance in the preservation of higher order central nervous system functions.

SUMMARY

Evidence is presented which indicates that protein molecules or their synthesis play a crucial role in the mechanisms which trigger REM sleep. It is suggested that such protein molecules may act as a "gate" or "signal" to bring forth a series of events, physiological and/or biochemical, which leads to what we have come to recognize as REM sleep. It is additionally suggested that REM sleep, through its accompanying upsurge of protein shynthesis or proteins availability, plays a dual role, depending on the stage of development of the organism. During the neonatal period it aids processes of development (Roffwarg et al., 1966), while in latter stages of life, it participates in guarding the integrity of the neural circuity which subserves processes of memory consolidation.

REFERENCES

Adam, K. and Oswald, I. Sleep is for tissue restoration. Journal of the Royal College of
Physicians, 11: 376-388, 1977.

Bloch, V. Interaction between post-trial reticular
stimulation and subsequent paradoxical sleep
in memory consolidation processes. In. R. R.
Drucker-Colin and J. L. McGaugh (Eds.) The
Neurobiology of Sleep and Memory. New York,
Academic Press, 1977, pp. 255-272.

Bloch, V. and Fishbein, W. Sleep and Psychological
function: Memory. In G. Lairy and P. Salzarulo
(Eds.) Experimental Study of Human Sleep:
Methodological Problems. Amsterdam: Elsevier,
1975, pp. 157-173.

Brodskii, V., Gusatinskii, V. N., Kogan, A. B. and
Nechaeva, N. V. Variations in the intensity
of ^{3}H-Leucine incorporation into proteins
during slow wave and paradoxical phases of
natural sleep in the cat associative cortex.
Dokl Akademic Nank SSSR 215: 748-750, 1974.

Drucker-Colin, R. R. The possible participation of
REM sleep in the regulation of cerebral excitability. Boletin de Estudios Médicos y Bio-
lógicos (Mex.) 28: 335-346, 1975.

Drucker-Colin, R. R. and Gutierrez, M. C. Effects
of forebrain lesions on release of proteins
from the midbrain reticular formation during
the sleep-wake cycle. Experimental Neurology,
52: 339-344, 1976.

Drucker-Colin, R. R. and Spanis, C. W. Is there a
sleep transmitter? Progress in Neurobiology,
6: 1-22, 1976.

Drucker-Colin, R. R. and Benitez, J. REM sleep
rebound during withdrawal from chronic amphetamine administration is blocked by chloramphenicol. Neuroscience Letters 6: 267-271, 1977.

Drucker-Colin, R. R., Spanis, C.W., Cotman, C. W. and
McGaugh, J. L. Changes in protein levels in
perfusates of freely moving cats: Relation to
behavioral state. Science, 187: 963-965, 1975.

Drucker-Colín, R. R., Zamora, J., Bernal-Pedraza, J. and Sosa, B. Modifications of REM sleep and associated phasic activities by protein synthesis inhibitors, in press.

Fishbein, W. and Gutwein, B. Paradoxical sleep and memory storage processes. Behavioral Biology, 19: 425-464, 1977.

Hobson, J. A., McCarley, R. W., Freedman, R. and Pivik, R. T. Time course of discharge rate changes by cat pontine brain stem neurons during the sleep cycle. Journal of Neurophysiology, 37: 1297-1309, 1974.

Johnson, T. C. and Luttges, M. N. The effects of maturation on in vitro protein synthesis by mouse cells. Journal of Neurochemistry, 13: 545-552, 1966.

Jouvet, M. The role of monoamines and acetylcholine in the regulation of the sleep-waking cycle. Ergebnisse der Physiologie, 64: 166-307, 1972.

Jouvet-Mounier, D., Astic, L. and Lacote, D. Ontogenesis of the states of sleep in rat, cat and guinea pig during the first post-natal month. Developmental Psychobiology, 2: 216-239, 1970.

Kitahama, K. and Valatx, J. L. Effects du chloramphenicol et duthimphenicol sur le sommeil de la souris. Comptes Rendus de la Societe de Biologie (Paris) 169: 1522-1525, 1975.

Magherini, P. C., Pompeiano, O. and Thoden, U. The neurochemical basis of REM sleep: a cholinergic mechanism responsible for rhythmic activation of the vestibulo-oculomotor system. Brain Research, 35: 565-569, 1971.

McGinty, D. and Sterman, M. B. Sleep suppression after basal forebrain lesions in the cat. Science, 160: 1253-1255, 1968.

Oswald, I. Human brain proteins, drugs and dreams. Nature (London), 223: 893-897, 1969.

Pegram, V., Hammond, D. and Bridgers, W.   The effects of protein synthesis inhibition on sleep in mice. Behavioral Biology, 9: 377-382, 1973.

Petitjean, F., Sastre, J. P., Bertrand, N., Cointy, C. and Jouvet, M.   Suppression du sommeil paradoxal par le chloramphenicol chez le chat. Absence d'affect du thiamphenicol. Comptes Rendus de la Societe de Biologie (Paris) 169: 1236-1239, 1975.

Roffwarg, H., Muzio, J. and Dement, W.   The ontogenetic development of the sleep-dream cycle in humans. Science, 152: 604-619, 1966.

Rojas-Ramirez, J. A., Aguilar-Jimenez, E., Posadas-Andrews, A., Bernal-Pedraza, J. G., and Drucker-Colin, R. R.   The effects of various protein synthesis inhibitors on the sleep-wake cycle of rats. Psychopharmacology, 53: 147-150, 1977.

Voronka, G. S., Demin, N. N. and Pezner, L. Z. Total protein content and quantity of basic proteins in neurons and neuroglia of the supraoptic and red nuclei of the rat brain in natural sleep and deprivation of rapid eye movement sleep. Dokl Akademic Nank SSSR, 198: 974-977, 1971.

GROWTH HORMONE SECRETION RELATED
TO THE SLEEP AND WAKING RHYTHM

YASURO TAKAHASHI

Department of Psychology
Tokyo Metropolitan Institute for Neurosciences
Fuchu City, Tokyo, Japan

Twenty-four-hour secretory patterns of all the
human anterior pituitary hormones and some of their
target organ hormones have been elucidated during
the past 10 years. The secretory patterns of these
hormones have the following characteristics: 1)
All the hormones are secreted in a episodic or
pulsatile manner. 2) 24-hr secretory pattern of
each hormone has a definite circadian variation
closely related to the sleep-waking cycle. The
nature of this relationship varies with the hormone
as mentioned later. 3) These rhythmic secretions
of the anterior pituitary hormones are regulated by
the central nervous system. This type of control
is designated as open loop control mechanisms which
are different from closed loop control mechanisms
regulated by feedback systems.

There are several types of relationship between
hormone secretory rhythm and sleep-waking cycle.
As for growth hormone (GH) and prolactin (PRL), the
relationship is direct and sleep-dependent. Their
enhanced secretion follows immediately the shift
of sleep period (Takahashi et al., 1968, 1974a;
Honda et al., 1969; Sassin et al., 1969a; 1973).
On the other hand, ACTH-cortisol secretion is not
sleep-dependent. The circadian variation can be
dissociated from sleep by acute sleep-waking reversal (Orth et al., 1967). Thus, ACTH-cortisol
secretion has an inherent circadian rhythm. All
the anterior pituitary hormones have either sleep-
dependency or inherent circadian rhythm and some
have both of them as summarized in Table 1.

Secretory patterns of PRL and luteinizing
hormone (LH) in puberty have a ultradian rhythm
closely related with REM-NREM sleep cycle (Parker
et al., 1974b; Boyar et al., 1972). There is a
close association of hormonal secretion with a
specific stage of sleep in some hormones. This is

Copyright © 1979 by Academic Press, Inc.
All rights of reproduction in any form reserved.
ISBN 0-12-222340-3

HUMAN ANTERIOR PITUITARY HORMONES	SLEEP DEPENDENCY	INHERENT CIRCADIAN RHYTHM
G H	PRESENT	ABSENT
P R L	PRESENT	ABSENT
L H (PUBERTY)	PRESENT	PARTLY PRESENT
L H (ADULT WOMEN, FOLLICULAR PHASE)	PRESENT	ABSENT
A C T H (CORTISOL)	ABSENT	PRESENT
F S H	ABSENT	ABSENT
T S H	PARTLY PRESENT	OBSCURE

TABLE I

SLEEP-DEPENDENCY AND INHERENT CIRCADIAN RHYTHM OF
HUMAN ANTERIOR PITUITARY HORMONE SECRETIONS

best exemplified by the relationship between GH secretion and slow wave sleep (Takahashi et al., 1968; Honda et al., 1969; Sassin et al., 1969a). The relationship between hormone secretion and sleep varies with age in some hormones. The sleep-related enhancement of LH secretion occurs only during puberty (Boyar et al., 1972). On the contrary, there is a significant decrease in plasma LH concentration during the first 3 hrs. after sleep onset in the early follicular phase of the menstrual cycle in adult women (Kapen et al., 1973).

Since we reported sleep-related enhancement of GH secretion in 1968 (Takahashi et al., 1968), this relationship has been studied in more detail than is available for any other anterior pituitary hormone. This paper deals with the relationship between GH secretion and sleep-waking cycle with special reference to slow wave sleep and wakefulness prior to sleep onset and deals with an animal model of human sleep-related GH secretion in dogs and refers to possible mechanisms underlying this phenomenon.

SLEEP-DEPENDENT GH SECRETION AND ITS CORRELATION WITH SLOW WAVE SLEEP

Under physiological conditions, GH is secreted during sleep, after meals, physical exercise and psychological stress. However, the highest peak of plasma GH concentrations in a 24-hr period always occurs during stage 3 and 4, i.e. slow wave sleep (SWS), shortly after the onset of nocturnal sleep (Fig. 1). The incidence of this phenomenon is more than 90% in normal subjects of both sexes at the age between 5 and 50 years. The GH secretory pattern in sleep is highly reproducible in the same individual.

When the time of sleep onset is shifted by 3-4 hrs, a GH peak occurs shortly after the shifted sleep onset as shown in Fig. 2 (Takahashi et al., 1968; Honda et al., 1969). Even a 12-hr reversal of the sleep waking-cycle is followed immediately by reversal of the pattern of GH secretion (Sassin et al., 1969a). When sleep is interrupted for 2-3 hrs. another GH peak appears after resumption of sleep (Fig. 2) (Takahashi et al., 1968; Honda et al., 1969). GH secretion occurs also during daytime naps (Karacan et al., 1974). Thus, sleep-related

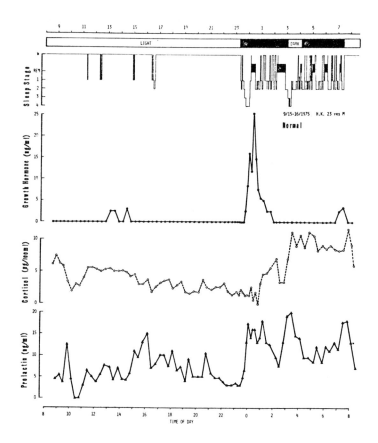

Fig. 1.   Twenty-four hour secretory patterns
of GH, cortisol and PRL with sleep stages in a
normal male subject at the age of 23 yrs. He was
fasted since the previous evening and sat in an
armchair in the daytime.

GH secretion shifts immediately with sleep onset
regardless of when sleep occurs, i.e. a sleep-
dependent phenomenon.
       The next question is whether this GH secretion
is associated with sleep onset per se or SWS, because there is high percentage of SWS in the first
2 hrs of sleep. Differential SWS deprivation
suppressed significantly, but not completely, sleep-
related enhancement of GH secretion (Sassin et al.,
1969b; Karacan et al., 1971). When the temporal

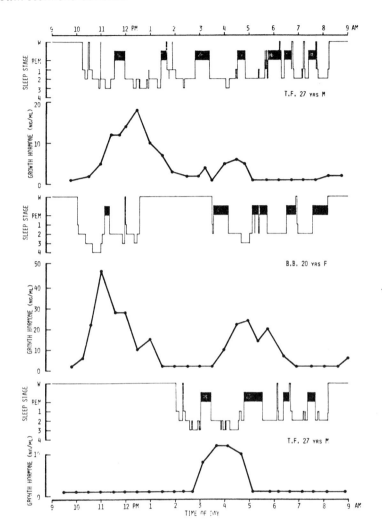

Fig. 2. Plasma GH levels and sleep stages during a night in normal subjects. From top to bottom are shown those during normal sleep, interrupted sleep and delayed sleep.

pattern of GH release at sleep onset was studied by frequent blood sampling at 4-min intervals, the first elevation of plasma GH level was not associated with the onset of stage 1 or 2, but was always preceded by high voltage delta activity (Pawel et al., 1972).

We studied in more detail the temporal relationship between SWS and GH secretion at sleep onset by frequent blood sampling and by power spectral
analysis of EEG frequency bands. In 4 normal male
subjects, ages 22-28 yrs. blood was sampled at 5-min
intervals for 60 min after the onset of stage 1 and
thereafter at 15-20 min intervals. Polygraphic
records were scored in 1-min epochs according to the
standardized criteria of Rechtschaffen and Kales
(1968). On the other hand, EEG's from C3/A2 and
C4/A1 derivations were recorded on a magnetic tape
and thereafter fed to a Walter-type EEG frequency
analyzer with power outputs. Ten-sec intensities
of power of 5 frequency bands, delta-2 (1-2 Hz),
delta-1 (2-4 Hz), theta (4-8 Hz), alpha (8-13 Hz)
and beta-1 (13-20 Hz), were continuously recorded
on 5 separate channels at a lower paper speed.
        Temporal relationships among sleep stages,
power spectra and plasma GH concentration were
examined on a graph as shown in Fig. 3. There was
a good correspondence between changes of stage 1
through 4 and increase in power intensities of delta
bands. In all the subjects, high voltage delta
activity of greater than 75 μv and slower than 2
Hz preceded the first elevation of plasma GH level
from the baseline by 5-12 min at sleep onset. This
finding is in agreement with that of Pawel et al.
(1972). Simultaneously with the first appearance
of high voltage delta activity, power intensities
of delta bands, especially of delta-2 band, increased
remarkably (Fig. 3). Although there was a close
temporal relationship between the initial rise of
plasma GH concentration and increased power intensities of delta bands, variation in GH levels subsequent to the initial rise was not always in parallel
with change in power intensities of delta bands.
As noted in Fig. 3, GH level began to rise immediately after the first SWS period of 2 min's duration
and continued to rise even during stage W, 1 and 2
which were interposed between the first and second
SWS periods in the first sleep cycle. In another
subject, GH level turned from a rise to a fall in
the middle of SWS period of 35 min's duration.
        These findings indicate that SWS or high
voltage delta activity, even if it was of short
duration, consistently preceded by several minutes
the first rise of GH level at sleep onset and that
GH release was related, not to duration, but to

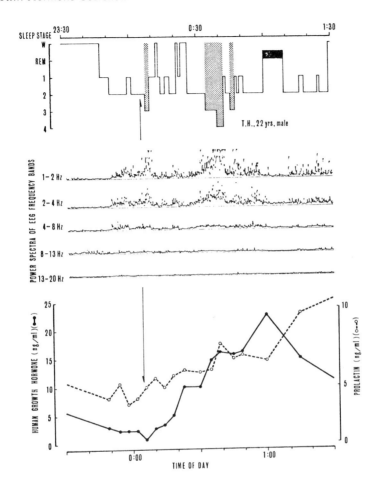

Fig. 3. Temporal relationships among sleep
stages, power spectra of 5 EEG bands and plasma
GH and PRL concentrations at nocturnal sleep onset
in a normal male subject at the age of 22 yrs. In
the upper figure, grey and black bars indicate SWS
and REM sleep periods, respectively, and an arrow
represents the first occurrence of high voltage
delta activity.

onset of SWS. This may explain the reason why
differential SWS deprivation could not completely
suppress GH secretion.

DISSOCIATION BETWEEN SLOW WAVE SLEEP AND GH SECRETION

It should be noted that SWS is not always associated with GH secretion. In normal subjects, GH
secretion is associated with SWS in the first and
sometimes second sleep cycles, but not often with
SWS in the subsequent cycles as shown in Fig. 1 and
2. There are a few normal adult women who do not
exhibit a GH peak at sleep onset in spite of their
normal sleep patterns including amount and distribution of SWS (Takahashi et al., 1968; 1976). It is
not until over the ages of 4-5 yrs. that a large
GH peak consistently occurs during SWS soon after
sleep onset (Illig et al., 1971; Finkelstein et al.,
1972). It is after the third month of life that GH
levels are significantly higher during sleep than
during waking (Vigneri and D'Agata, 1971). This
lack of adult-type sleep-related GH secretion in
infants may be explained either by immaturity of the
central nervous system connecting GH secretion with
SWS or by absence of monophasic sleep pattern as
discussed later. Absence of sleep-related GH secretion is often noted in aged normal subjects over
50 yrs. (Carlson et al., 1972; Finkelstein et al.,
1972). This may be explained partly by marked decrease of stage 4 sleep in the aged subjects.

Dissociation between GH secretion and SWS is
often noted in various pathological conditions and
in some drug administrations. Absence of a GH peak
associated with SWS at sleep onset has been reported in patients with acromegaly (Carlson et al.,
1972), Cushing's syndrome (Krieger and Glick, 1974),
hypopituitarism (Eastman and Lazarus, 1973), deprivation dwarfism (Powell et al., 1973), narcolepsy
(Takahashi et al., 1976), schizophrenia (Vigneri et
al., 1974), depression (Schilkrut et al., 1975) and
others. On the other hand, normal sleep-related
GH secretion has been reported in a majority of
cases with diabetes (Parker and Rossman, 1971),
hyperthyroidism (Dunleavy et al., 1974) and constitutional short stature (Illig et al., 1971; Eastman
and Lazarus, 1973).

This absence of sleep-related GH secretion in
patients with some endocrine and neuropsychiatric
disorders is rarely attributable to their abnormal
sleep patterns. It seems likely that various dys-
functions at level of the hypothalamus break non-
specifically the normal relationship between GH
secretion and sleep.

Narcolepsy is a unique sleep disorder: 1) day-time sleep attacks and disrupted nocturnal sleep break up the normal pattern of a single nocturnal sleep period and a single waking period, i.e. mono-phasic sleep pattern and 2) diurnal and nocturnal sleep usually begin with REM sleep, which is referred to as sleep-onset REM period.

We studied 24-hr secretory patterns of GH, PRL and cortisol in 4 male narcoleptic patients at the age between 30 and 34 yrs (Takahashi et al., 1977). Two of the 4 patients exhibited a GH peak concomitant with SWS after the sleep-onset REM period of noc-turnal sleep. In contrast to normal subjects, the peak value of GH concentration was not higher than those occurring either in the daytime or in the latter half of nocturnal sleep period. This may be considered to be related to the length of waking prior to the onset of nocturnal sleep as discussed later. The other 2 narcoleptics failed to have a GH peak at the onset of nocturnal sleep in spite of presence of SWS as illustrated in Fig. 4. All the patients had a sleep-onset REM period of 3-15 min's duration at the onset of nocturnal sleep. In none of them, GH release was detected during this sleep-onset REM period by frequent blood sampling. This absence of a GH peak at the sleep onset in the 2 patients could not be also explained by the presence of GH secretion in the daytime.

Sleep-related enhancement of PRL secretion was absent in one of the 4 patients. In contrast to the considerable intersubject variability in the patterns of GH and PRL secretion, almost normal circadian periodicity of plasma cortisol levels was present in all the narcoleptics. Comparison between the narcoleptic patients and the normal subjects in secretory patterns of GH, PRL and cortisol is shown in Fig. 5.

These differences in secretory pattern between GH, PRL and cortisol in the narcoleptic patients may be explained by different relationships between these hormonal systems and sleep: GH and PRL secretion depends directly on sleep and are altered in such a sleep disorder as narcolepsy while cortisol release is dependent on the inherent circadian rhythm and resistant to changes in sleep-waking pattern.

There are some drugs which suppress SWS-related GH secretion. As for psychotherapeutic drugs, oral

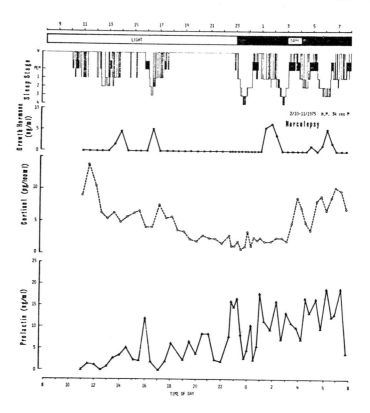

Fig. 4. 24-hr. secretory patterns of GH, cortisol and PRL with sleep stages in a male narcoleptic
patient at the age of 34 yrs. He was fasted since
the previous evening and sat in an armchair in the
daytime.

administration of chlorpromazine, phenobarbital,
isocarboxazid, diphenylhydantoin, chlordiazepoxide
(Takahashi et al., 1968) and flurazepam (Rubin et
al., 1973) did not suppress sleep-related GH secretion. Benzodiazepine derivatives, chlordiazepoxide
and flurazepam, reduced markedly stage 4 sleep, but
did not decrease GH secretion associated with SWS.
This may be explained by the above mentioned fact
that GH secretion is related not to duration, but
to onset of SWS.
        Sleep-related enhancement of GH secretion was
remarkably suppressed by oral administration of
imipramine (Takahashi et al., 1968). Although this

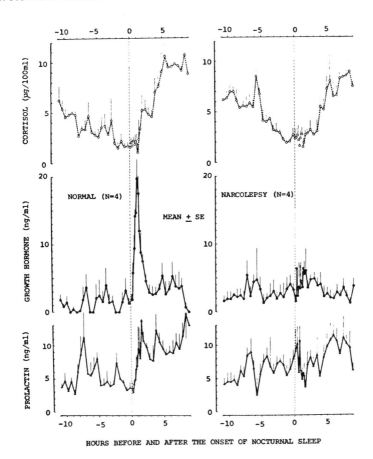

Fig. 5. The mean plasma levels ± SE of cortisol, GH and PRL in 4 normal male subjects (left) and 4 male narcoleptic patients (right) plotted as a function of time before and after the onset of nocturnal sleep.

drug markedly suppressed REM sleep, it did not affect SWS in early hours of sleep. Thus, this suppressive effect of imipramine on GH secretion is not due to SWS suppression. Recently, clomipramine infusion was reported to inhibit sleep-related GH secretion (Lacey et al., 1977). Oral amphetamine decreased slightly peak value of sleep-related GH secretion (Valverde-R. et al., 1976).

As to hormonal preparations, administration of
Zn-tetracosactrin (Evans et al., 1973), clomiphene
(Perlow et al., 1973) and medroxyprogesterone
(Lucke and Glick, 1971b) reduced sleep-related GH
secretion. Acute administration of hydrocortisone
failed to suppress nocturnal GH rise (Krieger et al.,
1972), but its chronic administration seems to
suppress it.

It is noteworthy that i.v. infusion of somatostatin or GH release inhibiting hormone completely
inhibited sleep-related GH secretion without
affecting sleep pattern (Parket et al., 1974a).
Thyrotropin releasing hormone, another hypothalamic
hormone, was reported to decrease sleep-related
enhancement of GH secretion (Chihara et al., 1977).

Dissociation of GH secretion from SWS can be
easily induced by administration of some drugs and
is sometimes seen in pathological conditions. Therefore, it is concluded that SWS and GH secretion are
closely related, but there is not a simple one to
one association or cause-effect relationship between
them. In other words, the mechanism controlling
GH secretion in sleep is not identical with that
producing SWS.

AN ANIMAL MODEL OF HUMAN SLEEP-RELATED
GH SECRETION IN DOGS

Although numerous papers concerning sleep-related GH secretion have appeared since 1968, almost
all of them have been restricted to human studies
and to descriptive ones. Animal studies are necessary for further elucidating the neuroendocrine control mechanisms of sleep-related GH secretion. There
are only a few papers dealing with the animal
studies: in baboons (Parker et al., 1972), rhesus
monkeys (Jacoby et al., 1974) and in rats (Willoughby
et al., 1976). In the chair-adapted baboon, GH
release in sleep similar to that in man was observed
whereas there was no apparent relationship between
sleep and GH secretion in the rhesus monkey and in
the rat.

An attempt was made to make a model of human
sleep-related GH secretion using dogs in our laboratory. Dogs were chosen for the reasons of their
blood volume sufficient for serial samplings, their

good adaptability to human handling and experimental environment, their similarities to humans in GH
response to various stimuli and availability of a
sensitive homologous double antibody radioimmuno-
assay for canine growth hormone (CGH) (Tsushima
et al., 1971) in our laboratory.

Our preliminary studies (Takahashi et al.,
1974b; 1975) reported that there was no close
temporal relationship between spontaneous CGH peaks
and sleep in a 24-hr period when a dog was left as
he was and that CGH secretion occurred concomitantly
with high voltage delta wave sleep shortly after
the onset of recovery sleep after 6-9 hrs. of
sustained forced wakefulness (FW). These findings
suggest that the length of sustained waking prior
to sleep onset is an important factor for revealing
a close relationship between sleep and GH secretion
in dogs as well as in humans.

Recent technical improvements have enabled us
to repeat 24-hr blood sampling with polygraphic
monitoring in the same dog: 1) blood transfusion
after experiments, 2) long-term indwelling of a
venous catheter without obstruction and 3) a device
for automatic enforced wakefulness. By this device,
sleep is automatically detected every 5 seconds
when 5-sec. integrated values of delta band of
cortical and hippocampal EEG exceed a preset level
and simultaneously 5-sec. integrated values of neck
EMG and body movements are below a preset level.
When sleep is detected, a sound as a conditioned
stimulus is given to the dog. If he is not awaken-
ed by this sound, an electroshock is given to his
neck to wake up as shown in Fig. 6. When this
avoidance conditioning is established, the device
easily keeps the dog awake as long as 12 hrs. without electroshocks. Enforced wakefulness can be
obtained by this method without exercise loading,
feeding and severe stress which may affect CGH
secretion.

The present study consisted of 2 series of
experiments. The purpose of the first one was to
compare the effect of this automatic FW on sleep-
related CGH secretion with that of manual FW and
to examine the effect of timing of 8-hr automatic
FW and the reproducibility of sleep-related CGH
secretion induced by this method. The second
series was studied for the purpose of comparing
the effects of length and timing of FW in the same
dog.

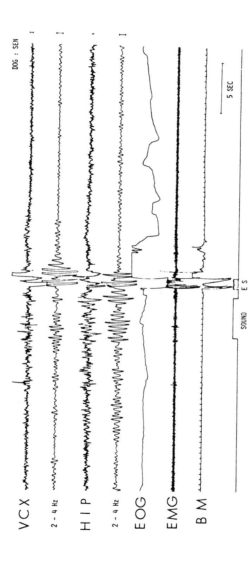

Fig. 6. Polygraphic tracing during enforced wakefulness induced automatically by the device described in thext in a dog.

Seven male mongrel dogs of adult age and 2 beagles aged 15-20 months were chronically implanted with electrodes for cortical and hippocampal EEG, EOG and neck EMG. A silicone catheter was inserted into the right atrium through the jugular vein and experiorized through the scalp to the top of skull. The dog was kept in a sound-attenuated, electrically shielded and temperature-humidity controlled chamber under a light-dark controlled condition˙(L:6:00-18:00, D:18:00-6:00). Sleep was polygraphically monitored and the records were scored in 1-min epochs into 4 stages: waking (W), light sleep (L), high voltage delta wave sleep (D) and REM sleep (REM). When more than half of the record consisted of high voltage delta activity in cortical and hippocampal EEG, it was scored as stage D.

One ml. of blood was drawn without disturbing the dog's sleep through a long tubing connected to the venous catheter from the outside of the chamber. Sampling intervals were 15 min. during 2 hrs. after FW periods and 30 min. for the rest of experimental periods. Blood samples were analyzed for plasma CGH and cortisol concentrations.

1. Spontaneous secretion patterns of CGH and cortisol concomitant with sleep stages were studied during a 24-hr. period in all the 9 dogs. They had polyphasic sleep patterns: sleep was frequently disrupted by awakenings shorter than 1 hr. in duration during the 24-hr. period. CGH peaks occurred 1 to 6 times over the 24-hr. period. It was difficult, however, to correlate these CGH peaks with sleep onset or any specific sleep stage. In none of the dogs, there was a circadian rhythm in cortisol secretion.

2. Eight-hr. FW was given to 8 dogs on 3 consecutive days: 1) manually from 9:00 to 17:00, 2) automatically from 9:00 to 17:00 and 3) automatically from 21:00 to 5:00. When a CGH peak occurred within 60 min. after the onset of recovery sleep following the FW period and its peak concentration was higher than 3 ng/ml above the baseline, it was defined as a sleep-related CGH peak.

Incidence and mean level $\pm$ SE sleep-related CGH peaks were shown in Table 2. There was no significant differences in incidence (Fisher exact probability test) and mean peak level (t-test) of sleep-related CGH peaks among these 3 days. Three of the 8 dogs had a sleep-related CGH peak on each

TABLE II

INCIDENCE AND MEAN LEVEL $\pm$ SE OF SLEEP-RELATED CGH
PEAKS INDUCED BY 8-hr MANUAL AND AUTOMATIC ENFORCED
WAKEFULNESS ON 3 CONSECUTIVE DAYS

ENFORCED WAKEFULNESS		SLEEP-RELATED CGH PEAK	
MODE	8-HOUR PERIOD	INCIDENCE	MEAN LEVEL (NG/ML)
MANUAL	9:00 - 17:00	5 / 8	10.1 $\pm$ 2.1
AUTOMATIC	9:00 - 17:00	6 / 8	9.7 $\pm$ 2.2
AUTOMATIC	21:00 - 5:00	7 / 8	9.4 $\pm$ 2.1

L : 6:00 - 18:00   D : 18:00 - 6:00   N = 8

of the 3 days. One example is given in Fig. 7.
     The sleep-related CGH peaks were associated
with stage D. High voltage delta activity almost
always preceded the initial rise of CGH level.
Stage L or REM of 1-2 min's duration sometimes
occurred during the 8-hr FW periods (Fig. 7). However,these short sleep period without high voltage
delta activity did not trigger CGH secretion. These
findings indicate that high voltage delta activity
at sleep onset triggers GH release in dogs as well
as in humans.
     Sleep-related CGH secretion was effectively
induced by the automatic 8-hr FW even if the timing
of FW period was shifted by 12 hrs. This means that
GH secretion at sleep onset is sleep-dependent not
only in humans, but also in dogs.
     3. Four dogs were subjected to automatic 8-hr
FW (9:00-17:00) on 5 consecutive days. Blood was
drawn on the last 3 days. Three of the 4 dogs
exhibited a sleep-related CGH peak on each of the
3 days as represented in Fig. 8. Another dog failed
to show it on the first day, but had it on the subsequent 2 days. The mean CGH peak level $\pm$ SE in
this series was 7.0$\pm$0.8 ng/ml. This result indicates
that sleep-related CGH secretion induced by the 8-hr.
automatic FW was highly reproducible (11/12=0.92).
     4. The last series of experiments consisted
of 5 sessions: 1) baseline day, 2) 3-hr. FW repeated

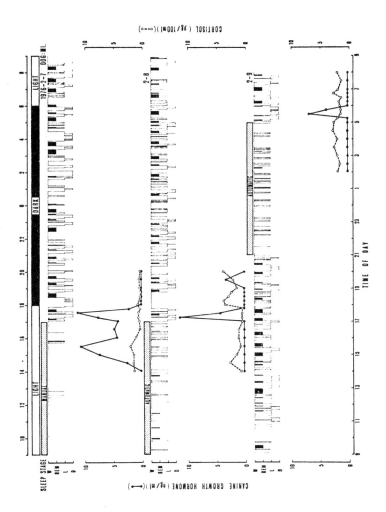

Fig. 7. Effects of 8-hr. forced wakefulness (FW) on CGH secretion in a dog. 24-hr. sleep-waking patterns and secretory patterns of CGH (solid line) and cortisol (broken line) are shown from top to bottom on 3 consecutive days of manual (9:00–17:00) and automatic (21:00–5:00) FW. Grey bars indicate FW periods.

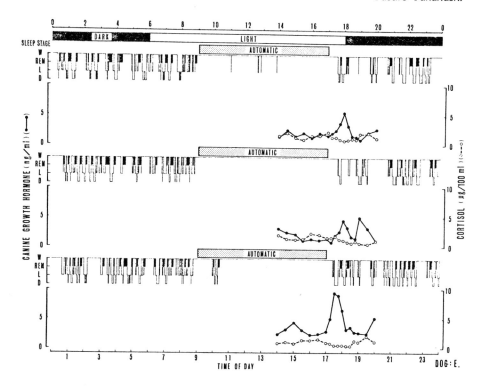

Fig. 8. Reproducibility of sleep-related GH
secretion induced by 8-hr. automatic enforced wakefulness (9:00 - 17:00) on 3 consecutive days.

at 3-hr. intervals 4 times a day, 3) 6-hr. FW performed at 6-hr. intervals twice a day, 4) 12-hr. FW
given from 21:00 to 9:00 and 5) 12-hr FW performed
from 9:00 to 21:00. Total FW time in a 24-hr. period
was 12 hrs. in each of these sessions. FW was automatically given to a dog for 5 consecutive days.
On the 5th day, blood was sampled and no electroshocks were given to avoid stress effect.

An example of this series was illustrated in
Fig. 9. Incidence and mean level ± SE of sleep-
related CGH peaks in this series were summarized in
Table 3. It is unlikely that difference in timing
of FW period affected the indicence of sleep-related
CGH peaks. Although the incidence increased with

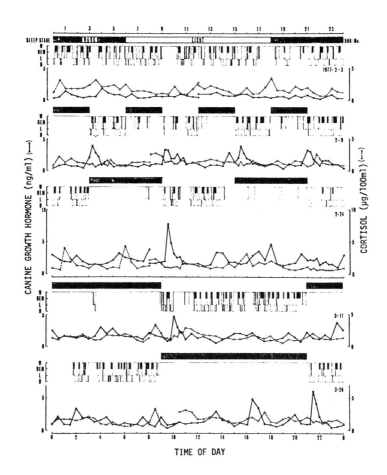

Fig. 9. Effects of 3-, 6- and 12-hr. forced
wakefulness (FW) on CGH secretion in a dog. 24-hr.
secretory patterns of CGH (solid line) and cortisol
(broken line) and sleep-waking patterns are shown,
from top to bottom, on baseline day, and 4 days
of 3-hr., 6-hr., reversed 12-hr. and 12-hr. FW.
Grey bars indicate FW periods.

the length of FW, the difference among the 4
sessions was not significant (Fisher test). There
were no significant differences in peak level of
sleep-related CGH secretion among the 4 sessions
except for the difference between the 3-hr. and 6-hr.
session (< 0.025, t-test).

TABLE 3

INCIDENCE AND MEAN LEVEL ± SE OF SLEEP-RELATED CGH
PEAKS INDUCED BY 3-, 6- AND 12-hr. AUTOMATIC
ENFORCED WAKEFULNESS ON SEPARATE 4 DAYS

ENFORCED WAKEFULNESS		SLEEP-RELATED CGH PEAK	
LENGTH (HRS)	TIME	INCIDENCE	MEAN LEVEL (NG/ML)
3	0:00 - 3:00 6:00 - 9:00 12:00 - 15:00 18:00 - 21:00	2/4 3/4 1/4 2/4 } 8/16	4.9 ± 0.8
6	3:00 - 9:00 15:00 - 21:00	3/4 3/4 } 6/8	7.8 ± 1.0
12	21:00 - 9:00	4 / 4	7.5 ± 2.5
12	9:00 - 21:00	4 / 4	6.7 ± 1.4

(between 3 and 6 length groups: < 0.025)

L : 6:00 - 18:00   D : 18:00 - 6:00   N = 4

Compared with the baseline day, mean total
sleep time and mean time spent in each sleep stage
were significantly reduced on the 4 days with FW
periods. Mean (±SE) reduction rate was $28.26 \pm 5.41\%$
in total sleep time, $49.13 \pm 7.39\%$ in stage L, $11.65 \pm 3.03\%$ in stage D and $34.56 \pm 4.25\%$ in stage REM in
the 4 dogs.

These results suggest that incidence of sleep-
related CGH peaks is independent of timing of FW
in a 24-hr. period and of the light-dark periods
and that it tends to increase with length of prior
FW, but its peak level do not necessarily increase
with the length.

Based on our observations in these dog studies
that the sleep-related CGH secretion induced by
enforced wakefulness was sleep-dependent and was
closely associated with high voltage delta sleep
at sleep onset, it seems reasonable to conclude
that this sleep-related CGH secretion is regarded
as a model of human sleep-related GH secretion. It

should be emphasized that adequate length of sustained wakefulness prior to sleep onset is an important factor responsible for uncovering a close
relationship between GH secretion and sleep in such
an animal as the dog who has polyphasic sleep
pattern.

POSSIBLE MECHANISMS UNDERLYING SLEEP-RELATED GH SECRETION

Based on accumulated evidences in many human
studies and in our dog studies, it is postulated
that two processes are essential to GH secretion as
related to SWS at sleep onset: 1) SWS as a trigger
mechanism and 2) sustained wakefulness prior to
sleep onset as a priming mechanism.

As already described, GH secretion is closely
associated with SWS in normal subjects. However,
this close relationship exists only in the first
sleep cycle and, moreover, at the onset of SWS.
There is no relationship between total amount of
SWS in the first 4 hrs. of sleep and amount of GH
secretion (Othmer et al., 1974). SWS or high
voltage delta activity consistently preceded by
several minutes the first elevation of GH level at
sleep onset.

These findings support the concept that some
priming or preparatory process for GH secretion is
already completed before sleep onset and that onset
of SWS triggers the GH secretory process.

If that is the case, what is the priming
process for sleep-related GH secretion? First,
pituitary reserve of GH which can respond to the
trigger-stimulus is essential. When GH has already
been released by such stimuli as stress just before
sleep onset, GH secretion may not occur in spite
of onset of SWS.

Now, we would like to claim that sustained
wakefulness prior to sleep onset closely related to
the priming mechanisms. During sustained quiet
waking, GH secretion is usually suppressed. When
sleep onset was delayed by 3-4 hrs. (Fig. 2)
(Takahashi et al., 1968; Honda et al., 1969) and
even by 8-9 hrs. (Sassin et al., 1969a), GH levels
remained at baseline level during waking at night.
When sleep was interrupted for 3-4 hrs., GH release
was suppressed during the intervening waking period
and another GH peak occurred shortly after resumption

of sleep as shown in Fig. 2 (Takahashi et al., 1968; Honda et al., 1969; Chihara et al., 1977). However, GH secretion did not occur after brief awakenings of shorter than 30 min. in sleep (Takahashi et al., 1968). Therefore, it is reasonably considered that sufficient length of prior wakefulness is necessary to sleep-related GH secretion. The finding that GH release was significantly greater during afternoon naps than during morning naps (Karacan et al., 1974) may be explained not only by different amount of SWS, but also different length of prior wakefulness.

The results of our dog studies add support to this concept. GH secretion occurs during SWS at the onset of recovery sleep after enforced wakefulness of longer than 3 hrs.

It is well know that SWS, especially stage 4, increases with length of prior wakefulness (Taub and Berger, 1973; Webb and Agnew, 1967). Thus, it seems reasonable to conclude that there is a functional correlation between SWS and prior wakefulness and, moreover, between sleep-related GH secretion and them.

It has been reported that physical exercise (Adamson et al., 1974), fasting (Parker et al., 1972) and hyperthyroidism (Dunleavy et al., 1974) increase sleep-related GH secretion as well as amount of SWS. Prior wakefulness may have the same effect. All these conditions increase demands on tissue reserves during waking. Since GH increases rate of protein and RNA synthesis, it is suggested that sleep-related GH secretion plays some reparative or restorative role in metabolic regulation. The observations mentioned above may give indirect evidences for this anabolic function of SWS-related GH secretion. In addition, the possibility that sleep-related GH secretion promotes somatic growth during period of physical development is included in the physiological significance of this phenomenon.

GH release from the pituitary is regulated by two hypothalamic hormones: GH releasing factor (GRF) and GH release inhibiting factor (GIF) or somatostatin. During quiet waking, either GIF may be released or GRF release may be inhibited at level of the hypothalamus since plasma GH concentration usually remains at baseline level. When SWS occurs after sleep onset, it may trigger GRF release in the hypothalamus, thus causing GH release from the

pituitary. Since the mechanism controlling GH
secretion is not identical with that producing SWS,
there must be some mediators between these two
mechanisms. There are accumulated evidences that
biogenic amines, such as noradrenaline, dopamine,
serotonin and acetylcholine, play important roles
in regulation of GH secretion (Müller, 1973) as well
as in sleep-waking mechanisms (Jouvet, 1972). Therefore, there is a high possibility that some neurotransmitters including biogenic amines are mediators
between SWS and GH secretion. Fig. 10 illustrates
a schematic representation of possible mechanisms
of sleep-related GH secretion as discussed above.

Effects of some drugs affecting actions of
biogenic amines on sleep-related GH secretion in
human normal subjects are summarized in Table 4.
There are some problems involved in these studies.
Since these drugs were administered orally, intra-
venously or intramuscularly, sites of action were
obscure. Many of these drugs have various actions
on the central nervous system other than those listed in this table. Accordingly, implication of
these results must be careful.

So far as we read the results in the table,
catecholaminergic systems may not be involved in
sleep-related GH secretion, because the drugs related
to adrenergic and dopaminergic systems such as l-
DOPA, chlorpromazine, phentolamine, propranolol and
isocarboxazid, do not affect it. On the other hand,
the effects of drugs with antiserotonergic action
are contradictory: cyproheptadine suppressed sleep-
related GH secretion whereas methysergide enhanced
it. It is noteworthy that all the 4 drugs with
anticholinergic action, methscoploamine, imipramine,
cyproheptadine and clomipramine as mentioned previously, have a marked suppressive effect on sleep-
related GH secretion. The suppressive effect of
these drugs is not attributable to changes in sleep
pattern because there was neither reduction in amount
of SWS nor change in the temporal distribution of
SWS.

It should be noted that the effects of the
drugs listed here on sleep-related GH secretion are
considerably different from those on GH response
to pharmacological provocative tests, such as
insulin and arginine infusion, in the daytime
(Mendelson et al., 1977). This implies that the
mechanisms underlying sleep-related GH secretion,

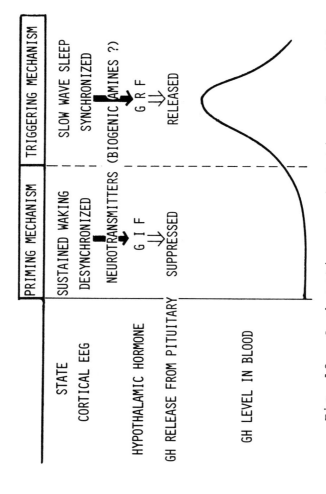

Fig. 10. A schematic representation of possible mechanisms of sleep-related GH secretion.

DRUGS	PHARMACOLOGY	DOSAGE	SLEEP-RELATED GH SECRETION	EFFECTS ON SLEEP SWS	REM	REPORTERS
L-DOPA	PRECURSOR OF DA & NA	400MG,IV 0.8-1.0MG/MIN	NO CHANGE	NO CHANGE	DECREASE	CHIHARA ET AL.(1967)
CHLORPROMAZINE	DA RECEPTOR BLOCKER	30MG, ORAL	NO CHANGE	NO CHANGE	INCREASE	TAKAHASHI ET AL.(1968)
PHENTOLAMINE	α-ADRENERGIC BLOCKER	5MG+0.5MG/MIN 3HRS,IV	NO CHANGE			LUCKE & GLICK (1971)
PROPRANOLOL	β-ADRENERGIC BLOCKER	1MG+0.06MG/KG/HR 2HRS,IV	NO CHANGE			LUCKE & GLICK (1971)
AMPHETAMINE	NA RELEASER	15MG,7DAYS,ORAL	DECREASE ?	NO CHANGE	DECREASE	VALVERDE-R ET AL.(1976)
ISOCARBOXAZID	MAO INHIBITOR	30MG,ORAL	NO CHANGE	NO CHANGE	NO CHANGE	TAKAHASHI ET AL.(1968)
METHSCOPOLAMINE	ANTICHOLINERGIC	0.5MG,IM	DECREADE	NO CHANGE	NO CHANGE	MENDELSON ET AL.(1976)
IMIPRAMINE	ANTICHOLINERGIC, NA REUPTAKE BLOCKER	50-75MG,ORAL	DECREASE	NO CHANGE	DECREASE	TAKAHASHI ET AL.(1968)
METHYSERGIDE	5-HT RECEPTOR BLOCKER	2MG/6HR,48HRS ORAL	INCREASE	NO CHANGE	DECREASE	MENDELSON ET AL.(1975)
CYPROHEPTADINE	5-HT ANTAGONIST, ANTIHISTAMINIC, ANTICHOLINERGIC	5MG/3HR,IV	DECREASE	INCREASE	DECREASE	CHIHARA ET AL.(1976)
MELATONIN		50MG/1HR,IV	INCREASE			CRAMER ET AL.(1976)

TABLE 4

EFFECTS OF SOME DRUGS AFFECTING ACTIONS OF BIOGENIC AMINES ON SLEEP-RELATED GH SECRETION, SLOW WAVE SLEEP AND REM SLEEP IN NORMAL HUMAN SUBJECTS

a physiological phenomenon, may be different from those of GH secretion induced by such artificial stimuli.   Although a clear-cut conclusion can not be drawn at present, it is likely that cholinergic and serotonergic mechanisms are involved in regulation of sleep-related GH secretion, but catecholaminergic mechanisms are not.   This problem is worth pursuing further.

SUMMARY

After a brief review of recent advance in research about relationship between human anterior pituitary hormone secretions and the sleep-waking cycle, the association of growth hormone secretion with the sleep and waking rhythm has been discussed in 4 chapters: 1) sleep-dependent GH secretion and its correlation with slow wave sleep, 2) dissociation between SWS and GH secretion, 3) an animal model of human sleep-related GH secretion in dogs and 4) possible mechanisms underlying sleep-related GH secretion.   It has been emphasized that GH secretion is closely related, not to duration, but to onset of SWS at sleep onset and this relation is sometimes dissociated in pathological conditions and in drug administrations and, in addition, that sustained wakefulness prior to sleep onset is essential to sleep-related GH secretion.   Our studies of a model of human sleep-related GH release in dogs have been described in some detail.   Finally, it has been postulated that prior wakefulness is a priming process of sleep-related GH secretion and SWS at sleep onset is its trigger process and that some biogenic amines are mediators between SWS and GH secretion.

ACKNOWLEDGMENT

The research presented in this paper was conducted in collaboration with Dr. Kiyohisa Takahashi, Dr. Teruhiko Higuchi, Mr. Shigemitsu Ebihara, Miss Yoshiko Nakamura, Dr. Yosizumi Niimi and Dr. Akio Miyasita and was supported in part by Grant in Aid for Special Project Research No. 212113 and by Grant in Aid for Scientific Research No. 137045 from the Ministry of Education of Japan.

REFERENCES

Adamson, L., Hunter, W. M., Ogunremi, O. O., Oswald, I. and Percy-Robb, I. W. Growth hormone increase during sleep after daytime exercise. Journal of Endocrinology, 62: 473-478, 1974.

Boyar, R., Finkelstein, J., Roffwarg, H., Kapen, S., Weitzman, E. and Hellman, L. Synchronization of augumented luteinizing hormone secretion with sleep during puberty. New England Journal of Medicine, 287: 582-586, 1972.

Carlson, H. E., Gillin, J. C., Gorden, P. and Snyder, F. Absence of sleep-related growth hormone peaks in aged normal subjects and in acromegaly. Journal of Clinical Endocrinology and Metabolism, 34: 1102-1105, 1972.

Chihara, K., Kato, Y., Maeda, K., Ohgo, S. and Imura, H. Suppressive effect of 1-DOPA on human prolactin release during sleep. Acta Endocrinologica, 81: 19-27, 1976.

Chihara, K., Kato., Y., Maeda, K., Matsukura, S. and Imura, H. Suppression by cyproheptadine of human growth hormone and cortisol secretion during sleep. The Journal of Clinical Investigation, 57: 1393-1402, 1976.

Chihara, K., Kato, Y., Maeda, K., Abe, H., Furumoto, M. and Imura, H. Effects of thyrotropin-releasing hormone on sleep and sleep-related growth hormone release in normal subjects. Journal of Clinical Endocrinology and Metabolism, 44: 1094-1100, 1977.

Dunleavy, D. L. F., Oswald, I., Brown, P. and Strong, J. A. Hyperthyroidism, sleep and growth hormone. Electroencephalography and Clinical Neurophysiology, 36: 259-263, 1974.

Eastman, C. J. and Lazarus, L. Growth hormone release during sleep in growth retarded children. Archives of Disease in Childhood, 48: 502-507, 1973.

Evans, J. I., Glass, D., Daly, J. R. and McLean,
    A. W. The effect of Zn-tetracosactrin on
    growth hormone release during sleep. Journal
    of Clinical Endocrinology and Metabolism,
    36: 36-41, 1973.

Finkelstein, J. W., Roffwarg, H. P., Boyar, R. M.,
    Kream, J. and Hellman, L. Age-relatee change
    in the twenty-four spontaneous secretion of
    growth hormone. Journal of Clinical Endocrino-
    logy and Metabolism, 35: 665-670, 1972.

Honda, Y., Takahashi, K., Takahashi, S., Azumi, K.,
    Irie, M., Tsushima, T. and Shizume, K. Growth
    hormone secretion during nocturnal sleep in
    normal subjects. Journal of Clinical Endocri-
    nology and Metabolism, 29: 20-29, 1969.

Illig, R., Stahl, M., Henrichs, I. and Hecker, A.
    Growth hormone release during slow-wave sleep.
    Helvetica Paediatrica Acta, 26: 655-672, 1971.

Jacoby, J. H., Sassin, J. F., Greenstein, M. and
    Weitzman, E. D. Patterns of spontaneous
    cortisol and growth hormone secretion in
    rhesus monkeys during the sleep-waking cycle.
    Neuroendocrinology, 14: 165-173, 1974.

Jouvet, M. The role of monoamines and acetylcholine
    containing neurons in the regulation of the
    sleep-waking cycle. In Ergebnisse der Physio-
    logie (Reviews of Physiology). Neurophysiology
    and neurochemistry of sleep and wakefulness.
    64: 166-307, 1972.

Kapen, S., Boyar, R., Perlow, M., Hellman, L. and
    Weitzman, E. D. Luteinizing hormone: changes
    in secretory pattern during sleep in adult
    women. Life Sciences, 13: 693-701, 1973.

Karacan, I., Rosenbloom, A. L., Williams, R. L.,
    Finley, W. W. and Hursch, C. J. Slow wave sleep
    deprivation in relation to plasma growth
    hormone concentration. Behavioral Neuro-
    psychiatry, 6: 67-70, 1974.

Krieger, D. T., Albin, J., Paget, S. and Glick, S. M. Failure of suppression of nocturnal growth hormone rise by acute corticosteroid administration. Hormone and Metabolic Research 4:, 463-466, 1972.

Krieger, D. T. and Glick, S. M. Sleep EEG stages and plasma growth hormone concentration in states of endogenous and exogenous hypercorti- solemia or ACTH elevation. Journal of Clinical Endocrinology and Metabolism, 39: 986-1000, 1974.

Lacey, J. H., Crisp, A. H., Groom, G. V. and Seldrup, J. The impact of clomipramine and its withdrawal on some nocturnal hormone profiles - a preliminary report. Postgraduate Medical Journal, 53 (Suppl. 4): 182-189, 1977.

Lucke, C. and Glick, S. M. Experimental modification of the sleep-induced peak of growth hormone secretion. Journal of Clinical Endocrinology and Metabolism, 32: 729-736, 1971 a.

Lucke, C. and Glick, S. M. Effect of medroxypro- gesterone acetate on the sleep induced peak of growth hormone secretion. Journal of Clinical Endocrinology and Metabolism, 33: 851-853, 1971 b.

Mendelson, W. B., Jacobs, L. S., Reichman, J. D., Othmer, E., Cryer, P. E., Trivedi, B. and Daughaday, W. H. Methysergide: suppression of sleep-related prolactin secretion and enhance- ment of sleep-related growth hormone secretion. The Journal of Clinical Investigation, 56: 690-697, 1975.

Mendelson, W. B., Jacobs, L. S., Sitaram, N., Wyatt, R. J. and Gillin, J. C. Methscopolamine: suppression of sleep-related growth hormone secretion and dissociation from slow wave sleep. Sleep Research, 5: 222, 1976.

Mendelson, W. B., Gillin, J. C. and Wyatt, R. J. Chapter 3: Neuroendocrinology and sleep. In, Human Sleep and Its Disorders. New York: Plenum Press, 1977, pp. 63-94.

Müller, E. E. Nervous control of growth hormone
    secretion. Neuroendocrinology, 11: 338-369,
    1973.

Othmer, E., Levine, W. R., Malarkey, W. B., Corvalan,
    J. C., Hayden-Otto, M. P., Fishman, P. M. and
    Daughaday, W. H. Body build and sleep-related
    growth hormone secretion. Hormone Research,
    5: 156-166, 1974.

Orth, D. N., Island, D. P. and Liddle, G. W.
    Experimental alteration of the circadian rhythm
    in plasma cortisol (17-OHCS) concentration in
    man. Journal of Clinical Endocrinology and
    Metabolism, 27: 549-555, 1967.

Parker, D. C. and Rossman, L. G. Sleep release of
    human growth hormone in treated juvenile
    diabetics: similarity to normal subjects and
    nonsuppression by hyperglycemia. Diabetes,
    20: 691-695, 1971.

Parker, D. C., Rossman, L. G. and VanderLaan, E. F.
    Persistence of rhythmic human growth hormone
    release during sleep in fasted and nonisocalori-
    cally fed normal subjects. Diabetes, 21: 241-
    252, 1972.

Parker, D. C., Morishima, M., Koerker, D. J., Gale,
    C. C. and Goodner, C. J. Pilot study of
    growth hormone release in sleep of the chair-
    adapted baboon: potential as model of human
    sleep release. Endocrinology, 91: 1462-
    1467, 1972.

Parker, D. C., Rossman, L. G., Siler, T. M., Rivier,
    J., Yen, S. S. C. and Guillemin, R. Inhibition
    of the sleep-related peak in physiologic human
    growth hormone release by somatostatin.
    Journal of Clinical Endocrinology and Meta-
    bolism, 38: 496-499, 1974 a.

Parker, D. C., Rossman, L. G. and VanderLaan, E. F.
    Relation of sleep-entrained human prolactin
    release to REM- NonREM cycles. Journal of
    Clinical Endocrinology and Metabolism, 38:
    646-651, 1974 b.

Pawel, M. A., Sassin, J. F. and Weitzman, E. D. The temporal relation between HGH release and sleep stage changes at nocturnal sleep onset in man. Life Sciences, 11:587-593, 1972.

Perlow, M., Sassin, J., Boyar, R., Hellman, L. and Weitzman, E. D. Reduction of growth hormone secretion following clomiphene administration. Metabolism, 22: 1269-1275, 1973.

Powell, G. F., Hopwood, N. J. and Barratt, E. S. Growth hormone studies before and during catch-up growth in a child with emotional deprivation and short stature. Journal of Clinical Endocrinology and Metabolism, 37: 674-679, 1973.

Rubin, R. T., Gouin, P. R., Arenander, A. T. and Poland, R. E. Human growth hormone release during sleep following prolonged flurazepam administration. Research Communications in Chemical Pathology and Pharmacology, 6: 331-334, 1973.

Sassin, J. F., Parker, D. C., Mace, J. W., Gotlin, R. W., Johnson, L. C. and Rossman, L. G. Human growth hormone release: relation to slow-wave sleep and sleep-waking cycles. Science, 165: 513-515, 1969 a.

Sassin, J. F., Parker, D. C., Johnson, L. C., Rossman, L. G., Mace, J. W. and Gotlin, R. W. Effects of slow wave sleep deprivation on human growth hormone release in sleep: preliminary study. Life Sciences, 8: 1299-1307, 1969 b.

Sassin, J. F., Frantz, A. G., Kapen, S. and Weitzman, E. D. The nocturnal rise of human prolactin is dependent on sleep. Journal of Clinical Endocrinology and Metabolism, 37: 436-440, 1973.

Schilkrut, R., Chandra, O., Oswald, M., Rüther, E., Baarfüsser, B. and Matussek, N. Growth hormone release during sleep and with thermal stimulation in depressed patients. Neuropsychobiology, 1: 70-79, 1975.

Takahashi, Y., Kipnis, D. M. and Daughaday, W. H.
    Growth hormone secretion during sleep. The
    Journal of Clinical Investigation, 47: 2079-
    2090, 1968.

Takahashi, Y. Growth hormone secretion during sleep.
    In M. Kawakami (Ed.), Biological Rhythms in
    Neuroendocrine Activity. Tokyo" Igaku-Shoin,
    1974 a, pp. 316-325.

Takahashi, Y., Takahashi, K., Kitahama, K. and
    Honda, Y. A model of human sleep-related
    release of growth hormone in dogs. Sleep
    Research, 3: 174, 1974 b.

Takahashi, Y., Takahashi, K., Higuchi, T., Inoue, K.
    and Honda, Y. A model of human sleep-related
    release of growth hormone in dogs: Twenty-four
    hour secretory patterns of canine growth hormone
    (CGH) and effects of 3, 6 and 9 hours of sleep
    deprivation. Sleep Research, 4: 288, 1975.

Takahashi, Y., Takahashi, K., Higuchi, T., Niimi, Y.,
    Miyasita, A. and Ishii, Y. Pituitary hormone
    secretions and narcolepsy. In C. Guilleminault,
    W. C. Dement and P. Passouant (Eds.), Narco-
    lepsy. New York: Spectrum Publications, 1976,
    pp. 543-563.

Takahashi, Y., Higuchi, T., Takahashi, K., Niimi, Y.
    and Miyasita, A. Twenty-four secretory patterns
    of growth hormone (GH), prolactin (PRL) and
    cortisol in REM narcoleptic patients. Sleep
    Research, 6: 89, 1977.

Taub, J. M. and Berger, R. J. Sleep stage patterns
    associated with acute shifts in the sleep-waking
    cycle. Electroencephalography and Clinical
    Neurophysiology, 35: 613-619, 1973.

Tsushima, T., Irie, M. and Sakuma, M. Radioimmuno-
    assay for canine growth hormone. Endocrinology,
    89: 685-693, 1971.

Valverde-R., C., Pastrana, L. S., Ruiz, J. A., Solis,
    H., Jurado, J. L., Sordo, C. M., Fernandez-
    Guardiola, A. and Maisterrena, J. A. Neuro-
    endocrine and electroencephalographic sleep
    changes due to acute amphetamine ingestion in
    human beings. Neuroendocrinology, 22: 57-71, 1976.

Vigneri, R. and D'Agata, R.   Growth hormone release during the first year of life in relation to sleep-wake periods.   Journal of Clinical Endocrinology and Metabolism, 33: 561-563, 1971.

Vigneri, R., Pezzino, V., Squatrito, S., Calandra, A. and Maricchiolo, M.   Sleep-associated growth hormone (GH) release in schizophrenia.   Neuroendocrinology, 14: 356-361, 1974.

Webb, W. B. and Agnew, H. W.   Sleep cycling within twenty-four hour periods.   Journal of Experimental Psychology, 74: 158-160, 1967.

Willoughby, J. O., Martin, J. B., Renaud, L. P. and Brazeau, P.   Pulsatile growth hormone release in the rat" failure to demonstrate a correlation with sleep phases.   Endocrinology, 98: 991-996, 1976.

NEUROPHARMACOLOGIC AND NEUROENDOCRINE
INTERRELATIONS OF HUMAN SLEEP

SOLIS, H., FERNANDEZ-GUARDIOLA, A. and VALVERDE-R., C.

Unidad de Investigaciones Cerebrales;
Instituto Nacional de Neurologia
and Departamento de Medicina Nuclear
y Clinica de Tiroides;
Instituto Nacional de la Nutricion
México, D. F.

INTRODUCTION

In the past decade a great deal of experimental
and clinical evidence has emerged suggesting that the
sleep-waking cycle and the secretory pattern exhibited by several anterior pituitary hormones in man,
represent two rhythmic neurohumoral efferences closely interrelated in time. However, available data
does not permit, to establish whether a causal relationship exists between the two phenomena, or if
they are independent, whether some common regulatory
signal (s) underlies their synchrony. In recent
years, our group has been engaged in a long range
project aimed at gathering information which may
help to understand the nature of such an interrela-
tion. Our studies include two basic approaches:
1. the pharmacologic manipulation of sleep-hormonal
related secretion, which provides indirect data on
the neural pathways and synaptic processes that may
be involved, and 2. the study of natural pathological endocrine models, which permits the assessment
of hormonal effects on the occurrence of the sleep-
stages.

This report summarizes part of our current work
and attempts to illustrate that the sleep-waking
cycle is a multifactorial neurohumoral process in
which neurotransmitters, hormones and some putative
peptidergic transmitters seem to interact in a
orderly fashion which thus gives rise to a major
integrative-homeostatic mechanism in the species.

Copyright © 1979 by Academic Press, Inc.
All rights of reproduction in any form reserved.
ISBN 0-12-222340-3

PHARMACOLOGIC MANIPULATION OF SLEEP-RELATED SECRETION

Although there is an extensive literature suggesting that central monoaminergic neurotransmitters participate in the modulation of the sleep-waking cycle and in anterior pituitary secretory activity (for reviews see Mendelson, Gillin and Wyatt, 1977; Valverde-R., et al., 1977), there is little available data on the assessment of both variables using pharmacologic agents that modify the metabolism, the release, and/or the central synaptic activity of such endogenous transmittters. This type of information seems necessary in order to systematically characterize the relationship between hormone secretion and sleep. However, as pointed out recently (Valverde-R., et al., 1977), the effects exerted by one particular central acting drug upon sleep-related secretion may differ and have to be distinguished from those observed on basal or "tonic" release, and from the acute or "phasic" hormonal discharge in response to several stimuli. Similarly, the type, dose, schedule, and pharmaceutical preparation of the administered drug, as well as its mechanism of action, needs to be considered. Furthermore, hormonal secretory patterns have to be distinguished between those corresponding to an endogenous circadian rhythm which, to a certain extent, are independent of the sleep-waking cycle (corticotropin, ACTH; and probably thyrotropin, TSH), from those that seem to be sleep-dependent or are nycterine rhythms (somatotropin, GH; prolactin, PrL; and probably gonadotropins, particularly LH). Available information derived from clinical studies in normal subjects is summarized in table 1. Data was grouped according to the primary mechanism of action of the drug used, and the three physiologic states - basal secretion, stimulated secretion and sleep related secretion - are distinguished. In this section of the paper, we will center our discussion on the clinical information derived from neuropharmacologic studies which evaluated the sleep-related secretion of GH, ACTH (by means of cortisol measurements), PrL, and TSH.

a.   Growth hormone

The sleep-related secretion of GH has been examined with more detail than for any other anterior pituitary hormone , and its association with slow-

TABLE I

Pharmacologic Manipulation of Central Aminergic Transmitters Acute Effects Upon Secretion of Some Anterior Pituitary Hormones in Normal Subjects *

Pharmacologic Agent	Basal Secretion[1]				Stimulated Secretion[1]				Sleep-Related Secretion[1,2]			
	GH	ACTH	PROL	TSH	GH	ACTH	PROL	TSH	GH	ACTH	PROL	TSH
Depleting Agents												
Reserpine			←		↓ Ins.							
Uptake Blockers												
Imipramine	→	→	←	←					→	→		→
Amphetamine	←	→		←	←	↑			→	→		→
Aminergic Releasers												
Amphetamine	←				←	↑			→			
Antagonistic Agents									CB-154			
Phentolamine (α)	→		↑		↓ Ins.-Arg.	Ins.		↑ TRH	→	→	↑	
Propranolol (β)	→		←	↑	↑ Ins.-Arg.	↑ Ins.		↓ TRH	↑	→	→	
Chlorpromazine (DA)	←	←		↑	↓ Ins.			↑ TRH	↑→	←	↑	
Ciproheptadine (5-HT)			←	→	↓ Ins.	↓ Metop. Ins.		↓ TRH				
Methysergide (5-HT)	←			↑	↓ Ins.							
Methergoline (5-HT)				↑	↑ Arg.	↓ Ins. Metop.	↑ Arg.					
Agonistic Agents												
Methoxamine, Clonidine (α)	→		→									
Isoproterenol (β)	←	←	→		↑ Ins.		↓ TRH	→ TRH				
Apomorfine (DA)	←			↑			↓ TRH	↓ TRH				
Br-ergocriptine (DA)	←	←	←	↑	↑ Ins.						↓	
Precursors												
L-Dopa								↓ TRH				
5-HTP												

* Acute applies for single to no more than a week administration of the drug. 1. See Valverde-R.C. et al 1977 for review of this literature.
2 See text for discussion and references. ↑ increase , ↓ decrease , → no effect.

wave sleep (SWS) seems well established, postulating
that previous wakefulness constitutes a "priming"
process and SWS acts as a "trigger" mechanisms
(see Takahashi this volume). Although sparse and
often conflicting, current neuropharmacologic data
suggests that, serotoninergic (5-HT), and/or cholinergic (Ach) pathways may participate in the GH
increase observed during sleep. However, full elu-
cidation of this complex control system, and the
nature of its relationship with sleep-regulatory
mechanisms, will not come easy.

   In contrast to the clear involvement of α and
β- adrenergic mechanisms (facilitatory and inhibitory respectively) on basal and phasic-GH secretion
during wakefulness, neither propanolol nor phentolamine infusion causes a significant effect on the
sleep-hormonal increase in humans (Lucke and Glick,
1971; Glick, 1971), or baboons (Parker, et al.,
1972). Furthermore, in these, as well as in other
sleep studies (Mendelson, Gillin, and Wyatt, 1977),
infusion of the B-blocker, propanolol, has no effect
on sleep pattern, whereas an α-blocker, thymoxamine,
increases REM sleep (Oswald et al., 1974). Similarly, chloropromazine, a dopaminergic antagonist
devoid of significant effect on sleep-profile when
administered in single oral doses of 100-150 mg
(Lester et al., 1971; Mendelson, Gillin and Wyatt,
1977), has no effect on GH-sleep secretion at a
single nocturnal dose of 30 mg (Takahashi, et al.,
1968). Furthermore, nocturnal infusion of L-dopa
(400 mg), significantly decreased time spent in REM
sleep, and had no effect on GH related discharge
(Chihara et al., 1976 a).

   On the contrary, imipramine (50 mg, single
nocturnal oral dose, Takahashi et al., 1968) inhibits,
and d-amphetamine (15 mg/day/7 days, spansule
morning oral administration, (Valverde-R., et al.,
1976) slightly reduces the sleep-GH related increase.
Both drugs have been found to suppress REM sleep and
enhance catecholaminergic activity by blocking
neuronal uptake of the transmitter at the synaptic
cleft. In addition, imipramine increases serotoninergic activity and exhibits central and peripheral
anticholinergic action, whereas amphetamine inhibits
Ach turnover rate in the striatum an effect probably
related to its ability to effectively block dopamine
(DA) reuptake (Cooper, Bloom, and Roth, 1974; Costa
et al., 1976; Diaz, 1976). Thus, it is possible

that through its anticholinergic activity both drugs
alter GH-sleep related secretion. This interpretation seems reinforced by recent findings showing
that methoscopolamine abolished and dissociated
from SWS, the sleep-related hormone discharge
(Mendelson et al., 1976).

However, recent preliminary data from our
laboratory (Valverde-R. et al., 1978), suggests
that chronic (10 years) abuse of amphetamine-like
drugs (including diethylpropion, 375 mg single
morning oral dose during the last 3 hr.), does not
disrupt nocturnal GH secretory profile and is
accompanied by an important increase of plasma
levels, which subside three to four days after
acute drug withdrawal. At this time the normal
sleep GH-related discharge was not observed (Fig. 1).
Similarly, comparative sleep recordings suggest
that schedule and time of drug administration do
exert different effects both qualitatively and
quantitatively (table 11). Similar GH-releasing
effects of amphetamines have been observed in man
after single intravenous administration of the drug
(methamphetamine 15 mg, Besser et al., 1969;
d-amphetamine 0.1 mg/kg b.w., Langer et al., 1975),
or in monkeys (Marantz et al., 1976), as well as in
man after chronic fenfluramine oral ingestion (Lewis
et al, 1971). Our findings may relate to the clinical observation of amphetamine tolerance and the
well-known withdrawal or rebound phenomena observed
after chronic ingestion of this type of drugs.
These observations, along with those that follow,
indicate the need for caution in interpreting results
of neuropharmacologic studies.

Theories on the involvement of serotoninergic
pathways in GH sleep related secretion are contradictory at present. Cyproheptadine a drug with
antiserotonin, antihistamine, and anticholinergic
properties (Douglas, 1975) does not suppress the
sleep related GH when infused (5 mg over a period
of 3 hr.) at the onset of sleep (Imura, et al., 1974).
However, using a similar dose and schedule (Chihara
et al., 1976 b), the drug blocked the GH-sleep
related increase in three out of seven subjects, and
when infused from 19.00 to 22.00 hr, it blocked or
delayed the release in the four unresponsive subjects.
Furthermore, in both schedules of administration,
SWS was significantly increased, whereas REM was
significantly reduced. Infusion from 04.00 to 07.00
hr, did not affect GH release during sleep, whereas

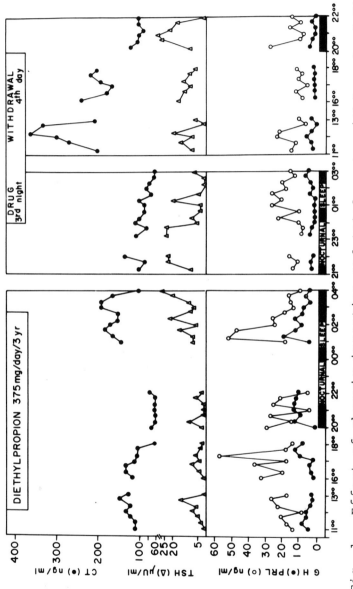

Fig. 1. Effect of chronic ingestion and total acute withdrawal of diethyl-propion on the secretory pattern of cortisol (CT), thyrotropin (TSH), prolactin (PrL) and growth hormone (GH) in a 24 year old female patient. Note that during drug ingestion the temporal profile seems preserved, suggesting a certain degree of tolerance to the drug (for further detail see text), Valverde et al., 1978. Unpublished results.

TABLE II

Hipnographic Changes Induced by Different Schedules of Amphetamine Ingestion *

Drugs Schedule (Dose, Preparation)	Sex Age	Total Sleep Time	Sleep Latency	W	Total Time Elapsed on Sleep Stages				
					1	2	3	4	REM
Control	F 18	356.0 (85.90)	25.3	58.4 (14.09)	9.9 (2.38)	164.5 (39.69)	27.9 (6.73)	73.9 (17.83)	79.9 (19.28)
d-Amphet. Single nocturnal dose (15 mg, spansule)		308.9 (81.52)	10.6	70.0 (18.47)	7.3 (1.92)	76.7 (20.24)	64.7 (17.0)	107.9 (28.47)	52.30 (13.80)
Control	F 19	415.8 (97.37)	11.3	11.3 (2.64)	14.6 (3.41)	179.3 (41.99)	20.6 (4.82)	84.4 (19.76)	116.9 (27.37)
d-Amphet. Daily morning dose (15 mg/7 d, spansule)		251.1 (59.78)	10.6	158.9 (40.21)	38.2 (9.09)	138.9 (33.07)	29.8 (9.09)	34.2 (8.14)	10.0 (2.38)
Chlorphentermine. Daily morning dose (30 mg/72 d, spansule)	F 18	388.6 (97.73)	1.66	8.8 (2.26)	24.6 (6.33)	198.5 (51.0)	66.3 (17.04)	—	90.5 (23.27)
Drug withdrawall (7th day)		415.4 (98.90)	2.2	4.6 (1.09)	8.3 (1.97)	181.6 (43.23)	72.5 (17.26)	—	153.0 (36.42)
Drug withdrawall (14th day)		411.9 (98.42)	3.4	7.3 (1.74)	15.3 (3.65)	175 (41.81)	46.5 (11.11)	9.3 (2.22)	165.8 (39.61)

* Data are expressed in minutes and (percentage) elapsed in each stage.
(Solís et al., 1978. Unpublished results).

REM sleep was significantly decreased. In contrast,
methysergide, a congener of LSD thought to have
central anti-5-HT activity (Douglas, 1975), decreases
the percentage of time spent in REM-sleep and increases GH levels during the first 2 hrs. of sleep
when administered at the total dose of 18 mg
(2 mg/6 hr, by mouth), the final dose being at 06.00
hrs and the sleep recording at 22.00 hrs (Mendelson
et al., 1975).

On the other hand, melatonin which has sleep-
inducing effects when administered in a single 1.25
mg/kg intravenous dose (Anton-Tay et al., 1971),
but not when administered under a chronic oral
schedule (1 mg/day/6 d, Fernandez-Guardiola and
Anton-Tay, 1974) has been shown to decrease latencies
for afternoon sleep onset and SWS, and to markedly
enhance peak GH secretion during SWS when infused
(50 mg) from 15.00 to 16.00 hrs (Cramer et al, 1976).
This result could be related to the increase of
serotonin levels in hypothalamus and midbrain
following administration of melatonin in rats (Anton-
Tay et al., 1968).

b. Cortisol

Data provided by neuropharmacologic manipulation of the sleep-waking cycle and assessment of
cortisol secretory pattern, seems to validate that
the fluctuations exhibited by the pituitary adrenal
axis represent a true endogenous circadian rhythm
less closely tied to sleep. Neither acute nor
chronic amphetamine ingestion supresses normal early
morning cortisol increase (Valverde-R, et al, 1976
and 1978) despite decreasing time spent in REM sleep
(Fig. 1). Furthermore, although recent studies by
Chihara et al, (1976 b), show that cyproheptadine
infused from 04.00 to 07.00 hrs (5 mg) blunted
cortisol increase and reduced REM sleep, the rest
of the schedules used by these authors did not
affect cortisol pattern despite the significant
reduction of REM sleep.

c. Prolactin

Although the effects of central active drugs on
daytime secretion of prolactin are widely studied,
only a few studies are concerned with analyzing
PrL sleep related secretion. Available information

suggests that DA transmission may be involved and
that PrL secretion is more closely associated to
REM sleep. Nocturnal infusion of L-Dopa (400 mg)
over a period of 6 hrs abolished PrL increase
(Imura et al, 1974). Similar results using the same
dose and schedule have been reported in extenso
(Chihara et al, 1976 a), indicating that besides
its PrL blocking effects the precursor significantly
reduced REM-sleep. Possible participation of dopaminergic mechanisms in PrL sleep related secretion
seems reinforced by the observation that thioridazine
(75 mg) increased the total nightly secretion of the
hormone (Kales et al, 1975). Recent preliminary
data from a single patient (Fig. 1) indicates that
chronic ingestion of amphetamine like drugs induces
a significant increase without affecting the nocturnal
discharge of PrL. Acute drug withdrawal was accompanied by a decrease to normal levels and the nocturnal rise was lost. A similar amphetamine induced
prolactin release has been reported after a single
intraperitoneal injection (1.2 mg) in the rat (Lu
and Meites, 1971), an effect that may be related to
the blocking action exerted by the drug on the DA-
neuron (Aghajanian and Bunney, 1974).
      Involvement of 5-HT is less clear. Studies
using methysertide (Mendelson et al, 1975) report
a highly significant decrease in sleep-related
secretion and suppression of PrL peak, as well as
reduction of REM-sleep. However, cyproheptadine
infusion (Chihara et al, 1976 a) does not alter
PrL secretion.

d.   Thyrotropin

      At present there is almost no data on the
effects of drugs on sleep-related TSH secretion.
The only available information comes from our laboratory (Valverde-R. et al, 1976) and shows that
amphetamine morning oral ingestion for seven days
(15 mg/day) blunted TSH normal nocturnal increase.
These findings were attributed to increased negative
feedback signal exerted by thyroid hormones at
pituitary level. Recent preliminary data (Valverde-
R. et al, 1978) indicates that subchronic (chlorphen-
termine, 30 mg/day, 72 days) or chronic (diethyl-
propion, 375 mg/day, 3 yr) morning ingestion of
amphetamine like drugs does not modify TSH nocturnal
release (Fig. 1), thus suggesting that a certain

tolerance may develop to the neuroendocrine effects
of this type of drug.

EFFECTS OF THYROLIBERIN (TRH) ON SLEEP-WAKING CYCLE

     Recently a great deal of attention has been
directed to the possibility that TRH may belong to
the new and growing family of putative peptide
neurotransmitters. This tripeptide widely distri-
buted in mammalian hypothalamic and extrahypotha-
lamic tissues (Vale et al, 1977), has been localized
in synaptosomal fractions (Barnea et al, 1977) and
when administered by microiontophoresis affects
neuronal firing rate (Dyer and Dyball, 1974; Wilber,
et al., 1976). Furthermore, TRH has been claimed
to be an effective antidepressant agent (Prange et
al, 1975), and exerts clear central stimulatory
effects counteracting the activity of several
depressant drugs (Breese et al, 1975; Brown and Vale,
1975; Horita et al, 1976; Cott et al, 1976).
     TRH action upon sleep has been explored in
three unrestrained chronically implanted cats by
continuous 24 hr recordings prior to and after a
single intravenous bolus of the peptide (150 μg),
Calvo et al, 1976). As depicted in figures 2 and
3, TRH administration elicited, during REM sleep,
a consistent increase in the total number of ponto-
geniculo occipital spikes (PGO). REM stages appeared
"fragmented" in a cyclic fashion, and therefore,
although their mean duration was not significantly
changed, their number and the total time spent on
REM sleep were increased. Waking stage (W) was
augmented in one animal 12 hr after TRH, whereas
the remaining two exhibited a discrete increase.
     Recent clinical studies (Solis et al, 1978)
comparing TRH (single i.v. nocturnal bolus, 500 μg),
d-amphetamine (single nocturnal oral dose, 15 mg),
and triiodothyronine (T$_3$ single nocturnal oral dose,
75 μg) effects on sleep pattern of normal volunteers,
suggest that the tripeptide and the drug exert similar qualitative effects. Both decreased total sleep
time and SWS, and increased W stage. However, TRH
did not affect stage 2 and REM sleep whereas amphetamine decreased both stages. Triiodothyronine
exhibited the opposite effects (table 3). These
results and similar recent findings using a different schedule of TRH administration (500 μg nocturnal

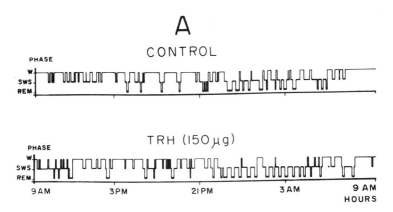

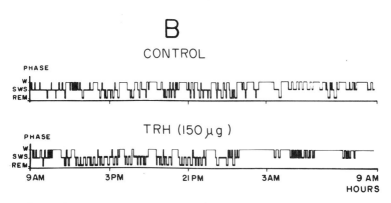

Fig. 2. Two examples (A, B) of qualitative
hypnographic changes observed after TRH 150 ug i.v.
administration in cat. Note that the number and the
total time spent on REM stage increased after THR
administration. In B, note also the remarkable time
spent in wakefulness (W) after TRH was given. W:
wakefulness, SWS: slow wave sleep, Rem: rapid eye
movements. (Calvo, et al, 1976, unpublished results).

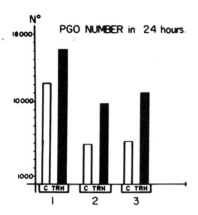

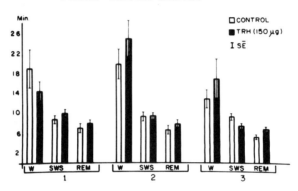

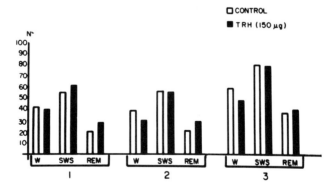

Fig. 3. Effect of I.V. injection of 150 μg TRH on PGO spikes and on sleep stages in 3 cats. From top to bottom note increase of PGO activity. Mean duration of sleep stages was not changed except for a significant enhancement of REM sleep in cat # 3. Also observe increased REM frequency after TRH administration.

Comparison of TRH, Amphetamine and T$_3$ Effects on Sleep Stages*

Experimental Condition		Total Sleep Time	Sleep Latency	Total Time Elapsed on Sleep Stages					
				W	1	2	3	4	REM
Phase (Control)	A	388.3 + 10.1 (92.93)	16.2	32.6 + 1.5 (7.08)	16.4 + 1.2 (3.95)	191.1 + 5.5 (46.07)	20.9 + 3.9 (5.02)	66.8 + 5.4 (15.83)	91.1 + 12.9 (21.79)
Phase (TRH)	B	340.1 + 11.5 (80.47)	11.7	74.8 + 10.9 (19.70)**	25.68 + 1.3 (6.8)	150.7 + 16.9 (35.8)	39.8 + 22.9 (9.48)	38.1 + 5.4 (9.06)**	89.4 + 11.0 (20.33)
Phase T$_3$	C	402.2 + 7.5 (97.19)	8.3	11.8 + 1.16 (2.80)***	12.9 + 1.7 (3.07)	197.3 + 2.8 (46.97)	45.5 + 4.2 (10.83)**	86. + 3.5 (20.48)**	96.0 + 10.4 (22.85)
Phase (d-amphetamine)	D	296.7 + 17.9 (70.6)	24	123.6 + 17.7 (29.4)	31.9 + 3.2 (6.8)	136.9 + 22.6 (31.7)	39.0 + 13.0 (9.1)	38.4 + 4.8 (10.5)	39.8 + 10.0 (9.5)

* Results expressed in minutes mean values + standard error, and (percentage) elapsed on each stage.
** p < 0.05, *** p < 0.01 compared to control. (Solfs et al, 1978).

bolus, followed by 1000 μg/3 hr infusion, Chihara
et al, 1977), may be consistent with the possibility
that the neuropeptide may be involved in the modulation of the sleep-waking cycle.

NEUROENDOCRINE MODELS

Since the initial all night sleep studies in
hypothyroid patients (Kales et al, 1967), the
possibility that hormones and some neuropeptides
may participate in the regulation of the sleep-
waking cycle has received little attention. The
possible participation of GH and other adenohypophyseal hormones has been proposed recently (see
Drucker-Colin in this volume). There is also
convincing evidence for the existence of sleep-
promoting neuropeptides (Schoenenberger and Monnier,
1977; Pappenheimer, 1977).
During the past few years some studies have
been conducted regarding the organization of sleep
stages during states of altered hormonal secretion
(Mendelson, Guillin and Wyatt, 1977). It is obvious
that those conditions presenting hormonal defi-
ciencies, as the myxedematous states due to primary
disfunction of the thyroid gland, or those secondary
to anterior pituitary failure, constitute the ideal
natural model to evaluate in a controlled and
graded manner the possible role played by hormones
in the sleep waking cycle.

a. Primary myxedema

The simultaneous longitudinal study of the
hypnographic and hormonal sleep-related secretions
in primary myxedematous patients (Martinez-Campos
et al, 1977; and Martinez-Campos, unpublished observations), suggests the involvement of thyroid hormones in the appropriate transfer of synaptic information and temporal organization of sleep and anterior pituitary synthetic secretory activities.
Absence of thyroid hormones is accompanied by completely disorganized sleep and hormonal secretory
patterns. Total sleep time is decreased and sleep
stage 1 and 2 occupy 80 to 100% of this time (proportion probably related to the chronicity of the
condition). Thus, SWS and REM are absent or

significantly reduced, whereas W is increased.
Concurrently, serum hormonal levels are low (except
TSH), there is no GH sleep related increase nor do
cortisol or PrL present their characteristic
rhythmicity. Replacement therapy (dessicated
thyroid) clearly reverses these abnormalities and
both sleep and hormonal profiles show a higher
degree of synchrony and organization.

b.   Secondary Myxedema

     A recent preliminary study in a 32 year old
female patient with postpartum pituitary necrosis
(Sheehan's syndrome) eleven years prior to the
study, was conducted to assess the effects of GH
and replacement therapy on the sleep-waking cycle
(Martinez-Campos et al, 1978). The study encom-
passed 129 days. A total dose of 24 U (4 μ/day/6
days) of human growth hormone (h-GH, clinical grade)
was administered before and after gradual sequential
hormonal replacement therapy that included dessicated thyroid (from 32 to 130 mg/day), cortisone
(20 mg/day), and estrogen (0.625 mg/day). As depicted in figure 4, results indicate that sleep stages
in Sheehan's syndrome are preserved although the
pattern is distorted. Administration of h-GH before
replacement therapy, abolished SWS and slightly
reduced REM sleep. After dessicated thyroid (32
mg/day/30 days) SWS reappeared, and six days later
h-GH administration induced a clear cut increase
in REM sleep. These results suggest that thyroid
hormones play a major role in mechanism (s) responsible for synchronizing sleep-stages and a permissive
one for GH effects on REM sleep.

CONCLUDING REMARKS

     Although still incomplete there are grounds for
optimism that a coherent network of pharmacologic
and neurohumoral information will develop in the
future that may help to understand in biochemical
and neurophysiological terms, what sleep is and
what its functions are. Up until now data has been
descriptive and has not yet provided mechanistic
explanations of sleep. However, it seems well
established (particularly for GH) that the neural

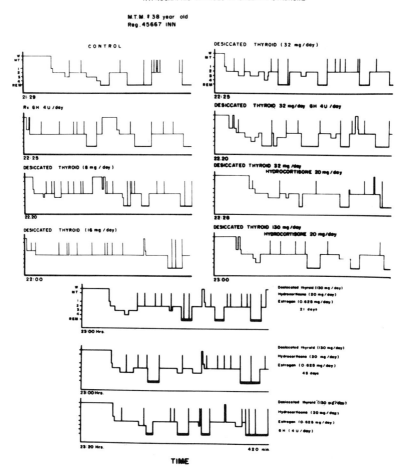

Fig. 4. Hypnographic sleep patterns in Sheehan syndrome before (control) and after gradual sequential hormonal replacement therapy (for further detail see text). (Martinez-Campos et al, 1978, unpublished results).

mechanisms involved in sleep-related secretion may differ from those controlling basal secretion and acute responses to several stimuli. Similarly, available data regarding neurohumoral influences on sleep suggest the possibility that endocrine secretions (particularly thyroid hormones and GH), as well as some neuropeptides (particularly TRH), may be involved in the regulation of sleep. Thus, based on this limited information and being aware of its fragility, we will offer a tentative explanations of the functions of sleep in the following paragraphs.

During wakefulness several cortical areas, particularly those involved in mentation and in the control and programming of voluntary movements, become activated. This activation, closely linked to constant environmental fluctuations, is characterized by its stochastic and random occurrence and subserves diverse control functions (Hernandez-Peon, 1955), which may be opposite and/or overcome several regulatory autonomic mechanisms, as shown for the pupilo-motor reflex and the orientation response (Fernandez-Guardiola, 1970). Thus, through corticofugal effects, the waking state seems to override and superimpose acute control signals upon some subcortical structures involved in autonomous regulatory processess, including the rhythmic and ever-changing sequence of regulatory events that characterize the hypothalamic-neuroendocrine pathways.

On the contrary, during sleep, such disruptive effects of wakefulness upon the "autonomic" hypoactivity seem to disappear. During sleep the subcortical structures oscillate, disengaged from the sudden and random "fight or fly" demands imposed by environmental conditions and physical activity through the activating reticular system and the anterior hypothalamus. Thus, sleep seems to subserve a major homeostatic function by "loosing free" those processes whose integration is dependent of a rhythmic sequence of regulatory mechanisms. Furthermore, the efficient operation and coordination of these regulatory neuroendocrine integrative systems requires pathways and signals (messages) that cannot be provided by conventional neurotransmitters alone. Thus, these systems utilize nonconventional neurohumoral messages such as classic hormonal feedback pathways and the putative peptidergic neurotransmitters which convey modulating influences to the entire system.

ACKNOWLEDGMENTS

We are grateful to our colleagues Drs. A. Martinez-Campos, J. L. Jurado, J. Maisterrena, and J. M. Calvo and the Staff from the Metabolic Ward for their collaboration in certain aspects of this work. Original work described in this paper has been supported in part by Grants from Centro Mexicano de Estudios en Farmacodependencia (CEMEF).
HGH, clinical grade was kindly donated by Proteic Hormones Distribution Program. Departamento de Investigacion y Medicina Experimental, IMSS. TRH was a generous gift of Hoechst de Mexico, S. A., and d-amphetamine and placebo capsules were kindly prepared by Smith-Kline and French.

REFERENCES

Aghajanian, G. K. and Bunney, B. S. Pre and post-synaptic feedback mechanisms in central dopaminergic neurons. In: P. Seeman and G. M. Brown (Eds.) Frontiers in Neurology and Neuroscience Research. Toronto, The University Toronto Press, 1974, pp. 4-11.

Anton-Tay, F., Chou, C., Anton, S., and Wurtman, R. J. Brain serotonin concentration. Elevation following intraperitoneal administration of melatonin. Science, 162: 277-278, 1968.

Anton-Tay, F., Diaz, J. L. and Fernandez-Guardiola, A. On the effects of melatonin upon human brain. Its possible therapeutic implications. Life Science, 10: 841-850, 1971.

Barnea, A., Oliver, C. and Porter, J. C. Sub-cellular compartmentalization of hypothalamic peptides: characteristics and ontogeny. Advances in Experimental Biology and Medicine, 87: 49-75, 1977.

Besser, G. M., Butler, P. W. P., Landon, J. and Rees, L. Influence of amphetamine on plasma cortico-steroid and growth hormone levels in man. British Medical Journal, 4: 528, 1969.

Breese, G. R., Catt, J. M., Cooper, B. R., Prange, A. J., Lipton, M. A. and Plotnikoff, N. P. Effects of thyrotropin-releasing hormone (TRH) on the actions of pentobarbital and other centrally acting drugs. Journal of Pharmacology and Experimental Therapeutics, 193: 11-22, 1975.

Brown, M. and Vale, W. Central nervous system effects of hypothalamic peptides. Endocrinology, 96: 1333-1336, 1975.

Calvo, J. M., Condes, M., Valverde-R., C. y Fernandez-Guardiola, A. Efecto de la hormona hipotalamica liberadora de tirotrofina (TRH) sobre el ciclo sueno-vigilia del gato. Boletin de Estudios Medicos y Biologicos, 29: 89, 1976.

Cott, J. M., Breese, R. G., Cooper, R. B., Barlow, S. T. and Prange, J. A., Jr. Investigations into the mechanism of reduction of ethanol sleep by thyrotropin-releasing hormone (TRH). Journal of Pharmacology and Experimental Therapeutics, 196: 594-604, 1976.

Chihara, K., Kato, Y., Maeda, K., Ohgo, S. and Imura, H. Suppressive effect of L-dopa on human prolactin release during sleep. Acta Endocrinologica, 81: 19, 1976 a.

Chihara, K., Kato, Y., Maeda, K., Matsukara, S., and Imura, H. Suppression by cyproheptadine of human growth hormone and cortisol secretion during sleep. Journal of Clinical Investigation, 57: 1393-1402, 1976 b.

Chihara, K., Kato, Y., Maeda, K., Abe, H., Furumoto, M., and Imura, H. Effects of thyrotropin-releasing hormone on sleep and sleep-related growth hormone release in normal subjects. Journal of Clinical Endocrinology and Metabolism, 44: 1094-1100, 1977.

Cooper, J. R., Bloom, F. E. and Roth, R. H. The Biochemical Basis of Neuropharmacology. Oxford University Press, 1974, pp. 146-701.

Costa, E., Cheney, D. L. and Recagni, G. Steady
    state and dynamics of putative neurotransmitters
    in teldiencephalic nuclei: a study using mul-
    tiple ion detection. In: P. B. Bradley and
    B. N. Dhawan (Eds.) Drugs and Central Synaptic
    Transmission. Baltimore, Ma., University Park
    Press, pp. 37-48, 1976.

Cramer, H., Bohme, W., Kendel, K. and Donnadieu, M.
    Freisetzung Von wachstumshormon und von
    melanozyten stimulie redem hormon im durch
    melatonin gebahnten Schlaf beim menschen.
    Arzneimittel Forschung, 26: 1076-1078, 1976.

Diaz, J. L. Correlaciones neuroquimicas de las
    alteraciones conductuales producidas por las
    anfetaminas. En: J. A. Maisterrena y C.
    Valverde-R. (Eds.) Las Anfetaminas. Cuadernos
    Cientificos CEMEF No. 6, pp. 131-157, 1976.

Douglas, W. W. Histamine and antihistamines;
    5-hydroxytriptamine and antagonists. In:
    Goodman, L. S. and Gilman, A. (Eds.) The
    Pharmacological Basis of Therapeutics. New
    York, MacMillan, 1975, pp. 590-629.

Dyer, T. G. and Dyball. Evidence for a direct
    effect of LRF and TRF on single unit activity
    in the rostral hypothalamus. Nature, 252:
    486-488, 1974.

Fernández-Guardiola, A. La voi visuelle chez le
    chat: Mecanismes de controle et de regulation.
    Boletin de Estudios Medicos y Biologicos,
    26:, 261-309, 1970.

Fernández-Guardiola, A. and Anton-Tay, F. Modula-
    tion of subcortical inhibitory mechanisms by
    melatonin. In: R. D. Myers and R. R.
    Drucker-Colin (Eds.) Neurohumoral Coding of
    Brain Function. New York, Plenum Press, 1974,
    pp. 273-287.

Hernández-Péon, R. Central mechanisms controlling
    conduction along central sensory pathways.
    Acta Neurologica Latinoamericana, 1: 256-264,
    1955.

Horita, A., Carino, M. A., and Chestnut, R. M. Influence of thyrotropin releasing hormone (TRH) on drug-induced narcosis and hypothernia in rabbits. Psychopharmacology, 49: 57-62, 1976.

Imura, H., Kato, Y., Hoshimoto, Y. and Nakai, Y. The role of biogenic amines in the regulation of pituitary hormone release in man with special reference to circadian rhythmicity. In: Kawakami, M. (Ed.) Biological Rhythms in Neuroendocrine Activity. Tokyo, Igaku Shorn, pp. 140-150, 1974.

Kales, A., Heuser, G., Jacobson, A., Kales, J. D., Hanley, J., Zweizing, J. R. and Paulson, M. J. All night sleep studies in hypothyroid patients before and after treatment. Journal of Clinical Endocrinology and Metabolism, 27: 1593, 1967.

Kales, A., Kales, J. S., Soldatos, C. R., Kotas, G, and Santon, R. Effects of thioridazine (Mellaril) on anterior pituitary secretion: changes in testosterone and prolactin. 2nd International Sleep Research Congress, Edinburgh, 1975.

Langer, G., Heinze, G., Reim, B. and Matussek, N. Growth hormone response to d-amphetamine in normal controls and in depressive patients. Neuroscience Letters, 1: 185-189, 1975.

Lewis, S. A., Oswald, I., Dunleavy, D. L. F. Chronic fenfluramine administration: Some cerebral effects. British Medical Journal 3:67-70, 1971

Lester, B. K., Coulter, J. D., Cowden, L. C. and Williams, H. L. Chlorpromazine and human sleep. Psychopharmacologia 20: 280-287, 1971.

Lu, K. H. and Meites, J. Inhibition by L-dopa and and monoamine oxidase inhibitors of pituitary prolactin release; stimulation by methyldopa and d-amphetamine. Proceedings of the Society of Experimental Biology and Medicine, 137: 480-483, 1971.

Lucke, C. and Glick, S.   Experimental modification
   of the sleep-induced peak for growth hormone
   secretion. Journal of Clinical Endocrinology
   and Metabolism, 32: 729-736, 1971.

Marants, R., Sachar, E. J., Weitzman, E. and Sassin,
   J.   Cortisol and GH response to D- and L-
   amphetamine in monkeys. Endocrinology, 99:
   459-465, 1976.

Martinez-Campos, A., Jurado, J. L., Solis, H.,
   Ruiz, A., Fernandez-Guardiola, A., Maisterrena,
   J. A. and Valverde-R., C.   Sleep pattern and
   adenohypophyseal hormonal secretory activity
   in a myxedematous patient. Revista de Investigacion Clinica (Mex.) 29: 239-244, 1977.

Martinez-Campos, A., Jurado, J. L., Solis, H.,
   Maisterrena, J. A., Fernandez-Guardiola, A. and
   Valverde-R. C.   Sleep pattern in Sheehan's
   syndrome. Effects of somatotropin and repla-
   cement therapy. Revista de Investigacion
   Clinica (Mex.) 30: 188, 1978.

Mendelson, W. B., Jacobs, L. S., Reichman, J. D.,
   Othmer, T., Cryer, P. T., Trivedi, B. and
   Daughaday, W. H.   Methysergide. Suppression
   of sleep-related prolactin secretion and enhancement of sleep-related growth hormone
   secretion. Journal of Clinical Investigation,
   56, 690-697, 1975.

Mendelson, W. B., Jacobs, L. S., Sitaram, S. R.,
   Wyatt, R. J. and Gillin, J. C.   Methscopolamine:
   suppression of sleep-related growth hormone
   secretion and dissociation from slow wave sleep.
   Sleep Research, 5: 222, 1976.

Mendelson, W. B., Gillin, J. C. and Wyatt, R. J.
   Human Sleep and its Disorders. New York
   Plenum Press, 1977, pp. 21-94.

Oswald, I., Adam, R., Allen, S., Burack, R., Spence
   M. and Thacore, V. Alpha adrenergic blocker,
   thymoxamine and mesoridazine both increase
   human REM sleep duration. Sleep Research, 3:
   62, 1974.

Parker, D. C., Morishima, M., Koerker, D. J., Gale, C. C. and Goodner, C. J. Pilot study of growth hormone release in the sleep of the chair adapted baboon: potential as model of human sleep release. Endocrinology, 91: 1462-1467, 1972.

Pappenheimer, J. R. The sleep factor. Scientific American, 235: 24-29, 1976.

Prange, A. J., Jr., Breese, G. R., Wilson, I. C. and Lipton, M. A. Pituitary and suprapituitary hormones: brain-behavioral effects. In: E. J. Sachar (Ed.) Topics in Psychoendocrinology. New York, Grune & Stratton, pp. 105-120, 1975.

Schoenenberger, G. and Monnier, M. The synthetic delta sleep inducing peptide (DSIP) Proceedings of the 27th International Congress of Physiological Science, Vol. 12, 678, 1977.

Solis, H., Jurado, J. L., Martinez-Campos, A., Maisterrena, J., Fernandez-Guardiola, A. and Valverde-R., C. Thyroliberin (TRH), D-amphetamine and triodo-thyronine (T3) effects on human sleep. Waking and Sleeping, in press, 1978.

Takahashi, Y., Kipnis, D. F. and Daughaday, W. H. Growth hormone secretion during sleep. Journal of Clinical Investigation, 47: 2079-2090, 1968.

Vale, W., Rivier, C. and Brown, M. Regulatory peptides of the hypothalamus. Annual Review of Physiology, 39: 473-528, 1977.

Valverde-R., C., Pastrana, L. S., Ruiz, J. A. Solis, H., Jurado, J. L., Sordo, C. M., Fernandez-Guardiola, A., and Maisterrena, J. A. Neuroendocrine and electroencephalographic sleep changes due to acute amphetamine ingestion in human beings. Neuroendocrinology, 22: 57-71, 1976.

Valverde-R., C., Martinez-Campos, A., Solis, H. and Jurado, J. L. Neurotrasmisores monoaminergicos, sueno y secreciones adenohipofisiarias en el hombre. Revista de Investigacion Clinica (Mex.) 29: 47-62, 1977.

Valverde-R., C., Martinez-Campos, A., Mora, B. R.,
    Ruiz, J. A., Solis, H., Jurado, J. L. and
    Maisterrena, J. A. Neuroendocrine effects of
    amphetamine abuse. Revista de Investigacion
    Clinica (Mex.) 30: 189, 1978.

Wilber, J. F., Montoya, E., Plotnikoff, N. P.,
    White, W. F., Gendrich, R., Renaud, L. and
    Maetin, J. B. Gonadotropin-releasing hormone
    and thyrotropin-releasing hormone: distribu-
    tion and effects in the central nervous
    system. Recent Progress in Hormone Research,
    32: 117-159, 1975.

ONTOGENETIC AND CLINICAL STUDIES OF SLEEP STATE
ORGANIZATION AND DISSOCIATION

DENNIS J. McGINTY

V. A. Hospital
Sepulveda, California

Developmental changes in the characteristics
of sleep provide us with a most dramatic experiment
of nature and, hopefully, a useful tool in searching for the functions of sleep. The early developmental period of mammals is associated with a qualitative and quantitative restructuring of sleep
state patterns. First, the distribution of sleep
into active sleep (AS)[1] and quiet sleep (QS)[1]
shifts from a predominance of AS to predominance of
QS (Cadilhac et al., 1962; Delange et al., 1962;
Monod et al., 1964; Roffwarg et al., 1966). Secondly, as emphasized originally by Monod et al. (1964)
and Parmelee et al. (1967) the QS and AS states
themselves exhibit internal reorganization. Indeed,
ontogeny is characterized by the gradual emergence
of distinct states from an undifferentiated pattern
of physiological organization and the gradual
recruitment of state-related characteristics in
cardiopulmonary, endocrine, and nervous system
functions. The present paper reviews these developmental changes and relates the emergent patterns
to experimental and clinical sleep state abnormalities. The concept to be considered is that adaptive
functions of sleep relate to the emergence of specific forms of nervous system organization that are
called states.

This paper will draw upon the results of
others as well as recent studies in our laboratory.
The experimental results presented here were
derived from standard polygraphic recordings from
10, 20 and 40 day old kitten groups. Healthy
kittens were surgically prepared with electrodes
and transducers for recording cortical EEG activity,
eye movements, neck electromyogram (EMG), respiratory patterns and the EKG. Most results were
based on analyses of 12-hour recordings carried
out in the presence of the mother and littermates,

Copyright © 1979 by Academic Press, Inc.
All rights of reproduction in any form reserved.
ISBN 0-12-222340-3

thus minimizing the effects of the laboratory environment. Methodological variations and analysis
techniques are described with the results. Detailed descriptions of our procedures are available
elsewhere (McGinty et al., 1977; Stevenson and
McGinty, 1978).

Sample polygraphic recordings are shown in
Fig. 1. Kittens of each age, including 10 day
kittens, exhibited epochs of three types of physiological patterns. According to well known conven-
tions, epochs of relative somatic quiescence are
labeled QS; epochs with phasic somatic events such
as eye movements and twitches, but without tonic
muscle activity, are labeled AS; and epochs with
tonic and phasic motor activity associated with
postural changes and other movements are called
waking (W). Specific criteria are applied to
determine the beginning and ending of each state
epoch. The records are divided into one minute
periods and each minute is classified as W, QS, AS
or mixed, according to the predominate state in
the minute. Based on the type of analysis, we
have determined the duration and proportions of
state epochs in each age group. As we will stress
below, measurement of sleep state percentages
neglects important developmental changes in intrinsic
state structure, but it reveals the developmental
shift in state distribution, as shown in Fig. 2.

Our results confirm previous studies, noted
in the introduction, showing that the proportion
of sleep classified as AS is greatly increased in
the newborn and infancy period, while the proportion of QS is reduced. Rat pups and kittens, which
are relatively immature at birth exhibit a greater
predominance of AS while the guinea pig, which is
relatively mature at birth, exhibits a higher proportion of QS (Jouvet-Mounier et al., 1970). The
full term human falls between these two extremes.
Recordings from guinea pigs in utero have shown
higher proportions of AS (Astic and Jouvet-Mounier,
1969). It is generally assumed that the relative
proportions of AS and QS reflect the degree of
maturity of the nervous system, although, as shown
below, other factors can also influence these proportions.

The fundamental and frequently-confirmed observation of AS predominance in neonates raises the

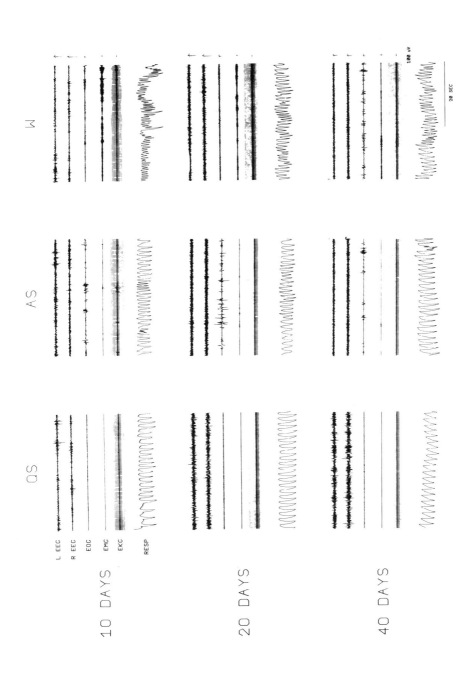

QS

AS

W

L EEG
R EEG
EOG
EMG
EKG
RESP

10 DAYS

20 DAYS

40 DAYS

100 uV

20 SEC

Fig. 1. Examples of polygraphic recordings during QS, AS and W from 10, 20, and 40-day-old kittens. The polygraphic data shown are left and right EEG, EOG, EMG, EKG, and respiration (inspiration down). Each age period is represented by 1 kitten. (From Stevenson and McGinty, 1978).

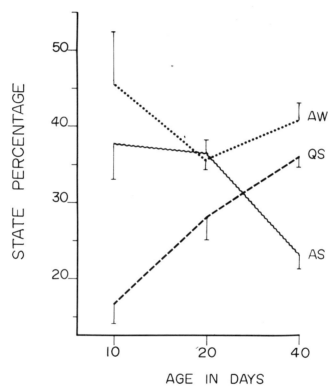

Fig. 2. Sleep-waking state distributions during kitten development. Mean state percentage and standard error in 10, 20, and 40-day kittens. QS increased at each successive age, whereas AS decreased after 20 days of age. Changes in W percentage were not significant. (From McGinty et al., 1977).

question of its functional significance. Does AS simply represent a primitive form of nervous system organization, a reflection of incomplete nervous

system capacity due to nervous system immaturity
(see below), or does the predominance of AS represent an instinctive adaptation which endows the
immature mammal with some capacity needed for
survival? For example, Roffwarg et al. (1966)
speculated that the AS provides endogenous nervous
system stimulation which plays a role in facilitat-
ing nervous system maturation. AS may also provide
the mammal with a capacity for inactivity and conservation of energy (McGinty and Siegel, 1978). Yet
a third concept is that AS predominance in a response to other physiological features of infancy
such as higher metabolic rate, protein synthesis,
or rapid nervous system growth. We cannot yet
solve this problem, but other observations will
help clarify the issues.

Development of State Organization

While it is true that both QS and AS can be
recognized in the 10 day old kitten the intrinsic
organization of sleep-state undergoes continuous
change during development and the adult forms of
these states are achieved gradually. This section
will outline these organizational changes. The
most immature human infants have been described by
Dreyfus-Brisac (1968). Previable infants between
24 and 26 W gestational age did not exhibit discriminable states changes. They were characterized
by continuous phasic motor activity and chin EMG
hypotonia and irregular respiration, suggestive of
active sleep. There was an absence of eye movements
and an unchanging EEG. In the newborn rabbit and
rat which are very immature at birth, a similar
physiological constellation has been observed, with
rapid eye movements appearing a few days post-
natally. In human infants at 28 to 30 weeks gestational age rapid eye movements become associated
with phasic movement and irregular respiration,
providing a picture of a more complete AS sleep
state.
Periods of quiescence are noted by 32 weeks
gestational age, but these periods are not necessarily associated with regular respiration and
absence of eye movements. The constellation of
parameters defining states in mature subjects is

achieved gradually. The developmental sequence of
concordance of state parameters can be quantified
by determining the percentage of epochs of motor
quiescence also exhibiting respiratory regularity
or absence of eye movement, or chin tonus, or
state-specific EEG patterns, or combinations of
3, 4 or 5 parameters. Table 1 from Parmelee and
Stern (1972) summarizes his results based on this
type of analysis on human infants. The variables
which are first useful in defining state are body
motility and eye-movements. Absence of movement

TABLE 1

A SCHEMATIC ORGANIZATION OF THE USEFULNESS OF
MEASURES IN DEFINING STATE
IN THE PREMATURE AND YOUNG INFANT

From Parmelee (1972)

	Weeks conceptional age					Months past term	
	24	28	32	36	40	3	8
Body Movements	+	+	++	+++	++++	++++	++++
Eye Movements		+	++	+++	++++	++++	++++
Respiration pattern			+	++	+++	++++	++++
EEG			+	++	+++	++++	++++
Chin EMG				+	+++	++++	++++

defines QS. Subsequently respiratory and EEG
patterns become reliable parameters, which tonic
EMG activity is last to discriminate state.
      We have carried out a related analysis in
kittens. We have compared various respiratory,
cardiac, somatic and EEG parameters of state epochs
which were defined by somatic variables.
Respiratory Patterns. Fig. 3 shows changes in QS

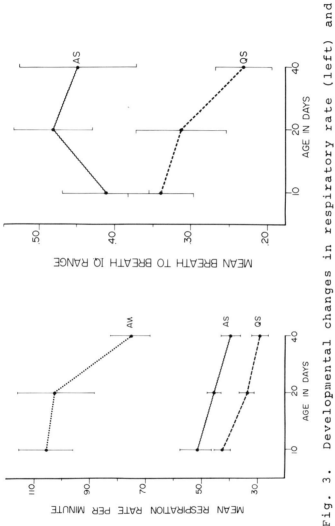

Fig. 3. Developmental changes in respiratory rate (left) and breath-to-breath variability (right) in relation to sleep states in the kitten. Ninety-five percent confidence limits for the means are shown (see text), from Stevenson and McGinty, 1977).

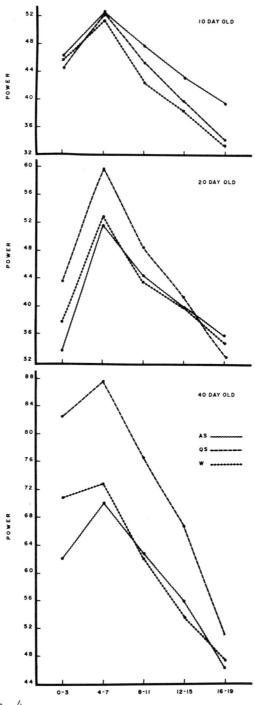

Fig. 4

and AS respiratory rate and variability during development. At 10 days of age a clear tonic difference between states was manifested in respiratory rate. Thus, a tonic excitatory influence on
respiration which changes with state was functional
in our youngest subjects. Since parallel developmental changes were seen in QS and AS rate, they
may reflect influences on breathing such as physical characteristics of lungs, that effect both
states equally. A different pattern was seen in
respiratory variability. With respect to this
parameter the states are initially similar, and
become differentiated. Respiratory variability
declined in QS, but was unchanged in AS. Variability in expiration time (te) rather than inspiration time (ti) accounted for state differences
(unpublished observations).

EEG. Visual inspection of the EEG did not reveal
difference between QS, and AS or W in 10 day
kittens. In 20 day kittens state differences were
often noticeable, but not consistent enough to be
useful in visual state scoring. At 40 days the QS
EEG exhibits the distinctive slow waves and spindle
that characterize adult SWS, while the W and AS
EEG appears to be the same. An analytic approach
to these data was carried using the tool of power
spectral analysis. Forty-five 16 second samples
from each state were obtained from 6 kittens in
each age group and analyzed by digital computer.
The spectral analysis was summed into five 4 Hz
bands which correspond to common verbal designation:
delta 0-3, theta 4-7, alpha 8-11, sigma 12-15, and
beta 16-19. The summed results are shown in Fig. 4.

Fig. 4. Power spectral analysis of EEG development in the kitten. The power in 5 frequency bands
from 12 minute samples of each state was summed
and averaged for 6 kittens at 10, 20, and 40 days
of age. Power in the 0-3 Hz band was reduced by
filtering. At 10 days (upper) AS was associated
with significantly higher power compared to waking
and QS in the 3 higher frequency bands. At 20
days QS power increases in the lower frequency
bands. AS and waking were no similar. At 40 days
QS differentiates further, particularly in lower
frequencies. AS differs from waking only in the
0-3 Hz band, (unpublished data from McGinty).

At 10 days of age overall spectral densities were generally similar in all states. Significant EEG differentiation was found only in AS. Power in the 12-19 Hz region was significantly elevated compared with QS and W, while the latter two states were indistinguishable. Young kittens are the only normal population reported to have similar EEG patterns in W and QS and distinct patterns in AS, but rats recovering from effects of large posterior hypothalamic lesions also shown EEG activation in AS before a change occurs in QS or W (McGinty, 1969, see below).

At 20 days there were small increases in power in QS in all frequency bands above the 0-3 range, such that QS was differentiated from W or AS. The latter states were indistinguishable at 20 days. Between 20 and 40 days power increased dramatically in all frequency bands and in all states. The increases are greatest in QS compared to W and AS. Therefore the difference between QS and other states became greater. W and AS remain indistinguishable.

Reflex Modulation. Adult AS is characterized by a power inhibition of spinal reflex transmission, in both extensor and flexor muscles, while reflexes involving antigravity muscles are facilitated in waking compared with QS (Pompeiano, 1967). The trigeminal monosynaptic massiteric reflex, which actives jaw closing massiter muscles, exhibits typical reflex suppression in AS and facilitation in W (Chase et al., 1968). The sequential development of masseteric reflex transmission in relation to sleep states has been assessed in kittens (see Fig. 5). In the 10 day kitten neither AS reflex inhibition or W reflex facilitation is observed. In fact, prior to about 20 days of age, opposite effects were seen. This result extends previous studies by Iwamura et al. (1967) and Chase (1971) which first showed absence of reflex inhibition in young kittens.

State Duration and Transitions. The preceding results have been concerned with the internal structure of sleep states. The duration of state epochs and the sequence of states also undergoes developmental changes. Epochs of all states become longer, due both to a reduction in the proportion

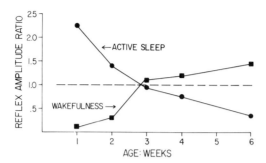

Fig. 5. Developmental changes in the relative amplitude of the masseteric reflex in sleep-waking states. Active sleep to quiet sleep and waking to quiet sleep amplitude ratios were found for each kitten and averaged in each group. Reflex depression in active sleep appeared at 4 weeks of age. In young kittens, changes opposite to the adult pattern were observed.

of short state epochs, and to an increase in the proportion of short state epochs, and to an increase in the proportion of long epochs. Fig. 6 shows the developmental change in proportion of long duration epochs of each state. The largest increase was found in the QS state. Thus, an increased capacity to sustain states of all types was associated with development of state organization.

We have also examined the patterns in transitions between each state and the subsequent state. In 10 day kittens the proportions of transitions types were not different from those which could be expected by chance. For example, the ratio of W-QS and W-AS was not different from the ratio of the number of epochs of QS and AS, the ratio of QS-AS and QS-W was different from the proportion of AS and W epochs, etc. Thus, transitions between states appear to be random. Fig. 7 shows the development of the relative proportion of W-QS and W-AS transitions. A chi-square test showed this distribution to be significantly different from

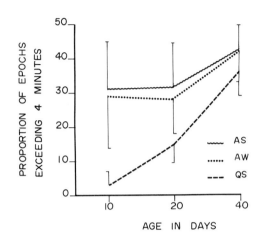

Fig. 6. Developmental change in epochs of
long duration (5 min.) Only changes in QS duration
were significant. The indicated measure of variability is the standard deviation. (From McGinty
et al., 1977).

chance in each 40 day subject. Other types of
transitions do not exhibit significant deviation
from proportions expected by chance at any age.

Summary: Developmental Perspective on Sleep.

        Table 2 indicates the sequence of entrainment
of behavioral and physiological patterns into QS
and AS, and emergence of temporal patterns in state,
as derived from the work of Dreyfus-Brisac (1968),
Parmelee et al. (1967), Hoppenbrouwers and Sterman
(1975), and Hellbrügge (1960), as well as our kitten
studies. "Early" parameters were state specific at
10 days of age in kittens and very premature
infants. "Intermediate" parameters began to distinguish state at about 10 days in kittens or at
32-36 weeks gestational age infants. "Late"
variables were not apparent until 20 days of age in
kittens or in full-term or slightly older human
infants.
        Developmental studies suggest that attention
be focused on the following features of sleep.

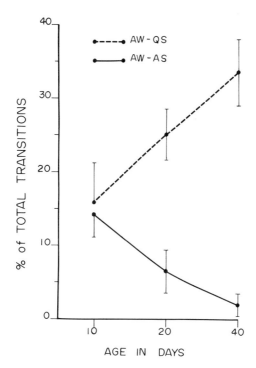

Fig. 7. Awake-sleep transitions. The relative proportions of W-QS transitions increased
whereas W-AS transtitions decreased during development. The W-QS transition became more predictable
than any other tranistion type. The standard
deviation of the samples is indicated by the
vertical line. (From McGinty et al., 1977).

    1. The phenomenon which has ontogenetically
and phylogenetically evolved is a "state," a recur-
ring constellation of physiological conditions. A
state is associated with a specific form of nervous
system organization (see below). Therefore, the
functions of sleep states should be related to the
properties of state-related organization in nervous
system processes. A specific organizational state
in the nervous system presumable endows the organism
with specialized capacities.
    2. Sleep state development is characterized
by gradual recruitment of coherent state patterns
in a specific sequence. Therefore, states are not

TABLE 2.   STATE ORGANIZATION SEQUENCE

Early

        behavioral quiescence - QS
        ultradian periodicity
        CNS excitation - AS

Middle

        respiratory variability declines - QS
        EEG high frequency augmentation - AS

Late

        EEG power augmentation - QS
        non-random transition probabilities
        sustained state epochs
        circadian rhythmicity
        reflex depression - AS

invariant, and elements of state may be dissociated. Many neurological disorders are best characterized as dissociated states (see below).

Sudden Infant Death

A focus of this symposium is to redefine the functions of sleep in the light of evidence that sleep amounts appear not to be related to essential waking functions. Not only is sleep difficult to relate to restorative processes, but sleep itself may precipitate life threatening events. The Sudden Infant Death Syndrome (SIDS) is an example of a sleep-related regulatory failure. Studies stimulated by interest in this syndrome provide additional insight into sleep functions.

SIDS is the leading cause of death in infants between 1 month and 1 year of age in modern western countries. It is characterized by sudden unexpected death in an apparently relatively healthy infant, for which no explanation has been found in intensive post-mortem examinations. SIDS most commonly occurs at 2 or 3 months of age rather than in the more fragile neonatal period. A large number of theories have been suggested and considered, many obvious explanations have been rejected, no explanation is widely accepted. Three well documented facts led

to our studies. 1. SIDS occurs during periods of
sleep and is silent (Bergman, 1970). 2. More
frequent or longer episodes of sleep apnea have
been observed in infants discovered to be cyanotic
while asleep but revived ("near miss" infants) or
in infants who were subsequently victims of SIDS
(Steinschneider, 1972). 3. Many victims of SIDS
exhibit a series of histological changes compared
to matched controls such as increased brown fat and
increased thickness of the smooth muscle wall of
pulmonary arterioles which indicates a history of
chronic hypoxemia (Naeye, 1973; 1974). For these
reasons SIDS victims have been compared to adult
sleep apnea syndrome patiens who exhibit hypoxemia
resulting from apnea specifically during sleep,
pulmonary hypertension, and who also are prone to
sudden death (Gastaut et al. 1966; Coccagna et al.,
1972).

Many approaches to the further analysis of
infant sleep apnea and respiratory control, and
characteristics of risk infants are under investigation throughout the world. We were involved in
the development of an animal model of normal and pathological sleep-related cardiorespiratory function in
infants which might be used for invasive experiments.
Given that many SIDS victims were chronically
hypoxic, we wondered how developmental changes in
sleep-related physiology might influence the adaptation to hpoxia. Accordingly, we monitored sleep
state, respiratory, and cardiac parameters in
kittens maintained in a hypoxic atmosphere (10% or
7% O_2) for 8 hours daily for either 3 or 8 days
(Baker and McGinty, 1977). Kitten groups were
exposed to the hypoxic conditioning such that the
final treatment day occúrred at 10, 20, or 40 days
of age.

Most kittens tolerated the hypoxic environment
without any obvious deteriorations of function.
These kittens exhibited increased respiratory rates
and decreased incidence of the stereotypic sleep
apnea episodes (see below) which caracterize normal
sleep. These changes represent compensatory adapta-
tions providing increased ventillation. A minority
of kittens were diagnosed as non-compensators because they exhibited slow irregular apneustic (long
end-inspiratory pauses) breathing (see Fig. 8) with
extreme heart rate variability. In some cases
breathing progressively slowed, turned into gasping

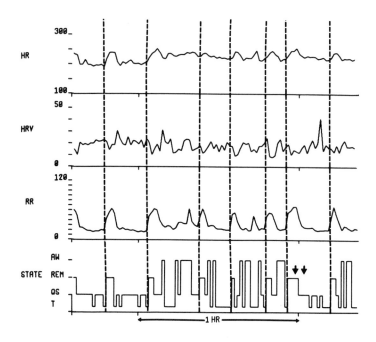

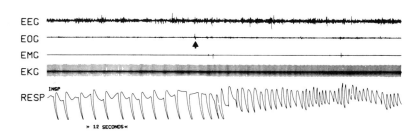

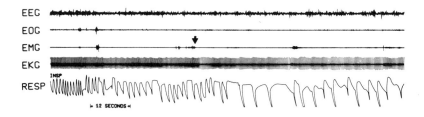

and finally stopped, leading to death. On special interest is the relationship of this failure syndrome to sleep-state patterns.

Characteristics of the failure syndrome are illustrated in Fig. 8. <u>Depressed breathing was observed exclusively in QS</u>. Transitions into AS were marked by an immediate normalization of respiration and augmentation and regularization of heart rate while AS-QS transitions resulted in resumption of slow breathing. Transitions to waking facilitated breathing in mildly effected animals, but not in extreme cases. Thus, the hypoxic respiratory failure syndrome was closely related to the QS state, while AS provided protection against respiratory depression.

Hypoxia had a second effect, namely, to augment the amount of QS at the expense of AS. Thus, the protective AS state was depressed by some consequence of reduced O_2 uptake, thus further increasing risk. Individual non-compensating animals, when compared to compensators, exhibited more extreme AS depression than other kittens of this age group. The single 40 day kitten which died exhibited less

Fig. 8. TOP. Computer plot of minute-by-minute heart rate (HR), heart rate variability (HRV), respiration rate (RR) and sleep-waking patterns recorded from a 10 day old kitten during the twelfth 2-hour hypoxia session. During QS, this 'non-compensator' exhibited extremely low RR (30 breaths per minute below controls) and slow HR (20-40 beats per minute below controls). RR and HR were clearly increased and HRV decreased by each AS epoch (AS onset is indicated by vertical broken lines). MIDDLE. Polygraphic recording of a 10 day old hypoxic kitten. AS onset, indicated by arrow marking first phasic eye movements (EOG), rapidly stimulated RR and HR. Slow apneustic breathing during QS is apparent in examples B, and C. BOTTOM. Termination of an AS epoch resulted in immediate respiratory slowing, bradycardia, and increased beat-to-beat irregularity in the EKG. The arrow marks the last phasic neck muscle activity associated with AS. (Modified from Baker and McGinty, 1977).

QS than all other 40 day subjects.

This study shows an important sleep state difference in adaptive physiology in infants. During AS breathing is maintained in spite of hypoxemia. We hypothesize that a critical epidemiological aspect of SIDS is explained by our observation. The increased incidence of SIDS in 2-3 month old infants compared with neonates, may result from the normal developmental increment in QS and decrement in AS. Any other factors increasing QS would also be expected to increase risk of respiratory failure.

Most non-compensating kittens (89%) were from 10 and 20 day age groups. Thus, QS in 40 day kittens is less dangerous than that in younger subjects. The crucial point is that immature QS differs from a more mature form with respect to resistance to respiratory depression. Obviously the respiratory system was capable of adequate function in younger kittens since it was readily achieved in AS. We believe that qualities of state organization must be examined to determine why immature QS fails to sustain adequate respiratory function. This study reminds us of an important concept related to functions of sleep states. Each state must possess nervous system processes adequate to maintain essential physiological functions such as breathing, cardiac output, water balance, and so on.

The concept that AS and QS are associated with different regulation processes is supported by more direct studies of respiratory control system. For example, Phillipson and Sullivan (1977) has described the additive effects of withdrawal of respiratory drives resulting from vagal afferents and peripheral and central chemoreceptors in chronic dogs breathing through intubated tracheal fistulas. During QS, combined withdrawal of these respiratory control processes resulted in almost complete cessation of breathing, while AS breathing was virtually unaffected by these procedures. In other words, AS breathing did not depend on any of the best-known respiratory stimulant mechanisms. Studies of temperature regulation have also shown important state differences. AS is associated with absence of temperature regulation (poikilothermy) while regulation was maintained in QS (Parmeggiani and Rabini, 1967; Parmeggiani and Sabattini, 1972;

Glotzback and Heller, 1976).

Another result of this study is the observation that infant sleep-state distribution is not exclusively a reflection of nervous system maturity. Increased QS can be produced by experimental manipulations such as hypoxia. This type of result was also illustrated in a previous study of environment and social deprivation of kittens (McGinty, 1971). Kittens were weaned at about 35 days of age and placed in completely enclosed cages for about 11 weeks; even exchange of food dishes of food dishes was done in the dark. Littermates were reared normally. Standard polygraphic recordings were then carried out both before and after isolated kittens were removed from cages and allowed to explore the laboratory for 24 hours. Compared to control kittens isolates exhibited increased QS and reduced AS prior to exposure to novely, but augmented AS afterwards. This result shows that differences between living in a complex world and impoverished world can influence sleep-state distribution. Since there were many differences between isolated and control kittens, specification of critical variables was not possible. However the study shows that state distribution in kittens is influenced by environmental factors as well as age.

Apneas and State Transitions. The significance of temporal aspects of state organization are illustrated in studies of respiratory pauses occurring during sleep, sleep apneas. Apneas attracted attention because of their relationship to pathogenisis in the Pickwickian syndrome. As noted above, sleep apneas have also been implicated in the etiology of SIDS. Sleep apneas also occur in normal infants and adults and the relationship between normal and pathological apneas is unclear. We have studied the incidence of sleep apneas in normal kittens, with particular emphasis on the relationship of apneic events to sleep organization. In the study apneas were defined as respiratory paused of 4.6 to 6.0 seconds (depending on age), a period equal to three times the average QS breath-to breath interval. A 6 second criterion is often applied to slower-breathing human infants. It must be emphasized that most apneas are beningn stereotyped events, frequently associated with a movement and following a deep breath (see Fig. 9A). Apneas

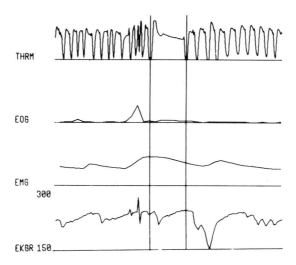

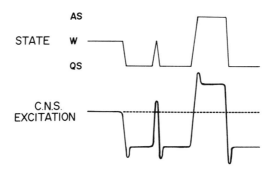

Fig. 9. UPPER. Heart rate and somatic activity associated with a typical AS-QS transition
apnea. Note typical irregular breathing in AS and
slow regular breathing in QS as detected by the
thermistor (THRM). The apnea was preceded by increased somatic (EMG) activity, a burst of eye movements (EOG), and an augmented breath. A sharp
heart rate (EKGR) decrement followed the apnea.
LOWER. Theoretical model explaining increased

in human infants have very similar properties.

Fig. 10A show the incidence of apnea in sleep-waking states in three kitten age groups. The highest apnea density was always greatest in transitional periods, least in waking. In some kittens the greatest number of apneas occurred in transitional periods, even though these periods comprise less than 20% of total time. In addition, these figures do not include apneas associated with brief interruptions of quiet sleep associated with movement. The latter may be transitional events, (QS-W-QS) but they did not meet our requirement for transitional periods. Thus, our figures may underestimate the number of transitional apneas.

Fig. 10B shows the distribution of transitional apneas according to types of state transitions. The highest apnea incidence was associated with AS-QS transitions, followed by W-QS transition in 20 and 40 day groups. The question is why do these types of state transitions yield high apnea densities. A possible explanation is shown schematically in Fig. 9B. According to this conception, a delay in resumption of breathing is most likely to occur at a state transition which is associated with a reduction in tonic nervous system excitability. Several variables, including neuronal unit activity and cerebral blood flow suggest that AS is a state of maximum nervous system excitation while QS is the state of least excitation. Nervous system excitation is moderately high in waking, although less than in AS. Thus, transitions from AS or W to QS are associated with diminished nervous system excitation. The model also implied that these transitions are associated with a transient "OFF" response like that seen in visual system with step reduction in illumination. The transient loss in non-specific excitatory drive on respiratory neurons is assumed to account for transient loss of rhythmic breathing.

apnea densities at W-QS and AS-QS transitions. The model assumes breathing is facilitated by central nervous system (CNS) excitation and that state transition decrements in CNS excitation are associated with a transient overshoot or "OFF" responses. This transient results in a temporary pause in respiratory drive.

   The implication of this analysis is that
periods of state transitions represent disjunctions
in regulatory processes.   Disjunctions may be understood as resulting from changes in tonic nervous
system activation, as hypothesized above.   There
may also be temporal gaps between offset of regulatory processes specific to the preceding state, and
onset of processes specific to the subsequent state.

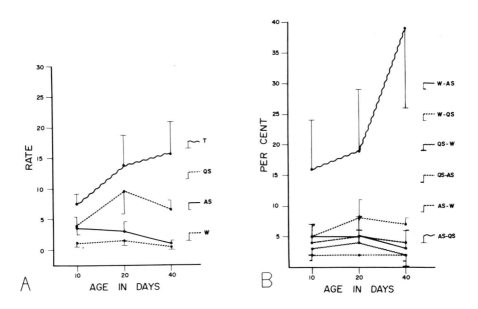

   Fig. 10.   (A).   Apneas densities per 100 minutes
of each state in normal 10, 20, and 40 day old
kittens.   Apnea density was greatest at state transitions, least in waking.   Quiet sleep (QS) exceeded
active sleep (AS) density at 20 and 40 days.   (B).
The percentage of state transitions of each type
associated with apnea.   AS-QS transition were most
likely to be associated with apnea at all ages.

Respiration is not the only process exhibiting reduced control at state transitions. Cadilhac et al. (1973) have noted that petit-mal epileptic paroxysms often emerge at transitions from waking to sleep while transitions from SWS to REM may be associated with convulsive seizures. Transient arousal from SWS may also trigger cardiac arrhythmias (Willens et al., 1972). It is note-worthy that neuronal units in the motor cortex (pyramidal tract neurons) exhibit divergent changes in unit discharge rate only during transient arousal from SWS (Steriade et al., 1974). I believe that future studies will reveal additional regulatory lapses during state transitions.

Dissociations in Adult Sleep

Consideration of sleep from a developmental perspective has focused our attention on organiza-tional aspects of sleep states including the emergence of sustained episodes of coherent con-figurations of specific physiological parameter patterns as seen in the normal adult. The useful-ness of this perspective is illustrated by a consi-deration of certain experimental and clinical sleep disorders, as well as sleep patterns in abnormal populations. Several examples are listed below.
1. Motor Behavior During Sleep. The most dramatic type of motor behavior during sleep is sleep-waking. Typically a child will sit up abruptly with a blank expression, move out of bed and walk rather clumsily, and be generally unresponsive to the environment and not attempt to communicate. However, obstacles in the environment are generally avoided. Sleep-walkers are aroused only with great difficulty, and they have amnesia for the episode. The incidence of sleep-walking is reported to be about 15% of children between the ages of 5 and 12 years. While it was expected that sleep-walking would be asso-ciated with REMS, a reflection of dreaming, this proved to be wrong. Jacobson et al. (1965) showed through polygraphic recordings (the subjects were connected through long mobile cables) that sleep-walking was associated with sleep stages III and IV including the presence of high voltage rhythm paroxysmal delta waves. These delta waves were found in most 6-11 month old infants, but may be a sign of immaturity in older children. In other

respects the nightly sleep cycle of sleep-walkers
was normal. Other less dramatic forms of motor
activity are also during sleep. These include
nocturnal myoclonus, tooth grinding and scratching.
These behaviors differ from sleep-walking in that
they are prevalent in stages II sleep and REMS as
well as stage III and IV. These studies suggest
that the normal association of SWS and behavioral
inactivity is the reflection of the coordinated
function of two distinct processes. Sleep may
occur without inactivity.

2. Waking With Atonia. The cataplexy that is
associated with the narcolepsy syndrome is characterized by precipitous loss of supporting muscle tone
which varies in intensity from fleeting sensations
of weakness and knee buckling and sagging of the
jaw to total collapse lasting many minutes (Yoss
and Daly, 1957). The episodes are frequently
triggered by emotions such as fear or laughter or
by stress. During an extended cataplectic attack and
victim is paralyzed and unable to talk, but he may
be able to move his eyes and understand communication from others. Therefore, the absence of perception which normally defines sleep is not present.
The cataplexic attack appears to be based on the
same motor inhibitory mechanisms that underlies
atonia in REM sleep, since the narcoleptic has a
strong disposition for sleep-onset REM, cataplctic
episodes have several specific motor system characteristics in common with REM periods, and symptoms
of deep paralysis and hypnagogic hallucinations are
best understood as sleep onset REM periods
(Rechtschaffen et al., 1963; Dement et al., 1966).
Thus, atonia normally associated with REM occurs
during waking.

3. REM without Atonia. REM sleep episodes associated with increased muscle tone and movement
including head elevation and swaying, hind limb
stepping movements, and even sporadic bursts of
rage-like behavior have been reported by Jouvet
(1962), Henley and Morrison (1974), and Jones et
al. (1977). This phenomenon is produced by lesions
of the dorsal pontine tegmentation, in or adjacent
to the locus coeruleus. The cats appear to be
exhibiting organized movement, but are unresponsive
to external visual or tactile stimulation. The
interpretation that these episodes correspond to
REM periods, in spite of the absence of atonia, is

based on observations that 1) the cats appear to be
asleep as evidenced by miotic pupils, relaxed
nictitating membranes, while awakening is associated
pupilar dilation, retracting of nictitating membranes, orientation to visual stimuli, and more coordinated movements, 2) other REM variables such as EEG
desynchronization and PGO waves and rapid eye movement are associated with the episodes, 3) the episodes follow SWS like normal REM periods and 4),
the waxing and waning of movements closely parallels
the pattern of twitching and quiescence of normal
REM periods. A related phenomenon has been reported
by Mouret (1975) in humans affected with Parkinson's
disease. Submental EMG activity persisted or developed during REMS episoded in 7 of 13 patients
studied. It is notable that Parkinson's disease
is associated with degeneration of the locus
coeruleus as well as the nigral-stratal dopamine
system (Foix, 1921).

4. Waking With REMS Phasic Activity. The PGO
wave is a phasic slow wave event that is usually
studied in the cats although analogous events appear
to be seen in the rat, monkey and man. Eye movement potentials, bear a general similarity to PGO
waves (Jeannerod and Sakai, 1970), but the REM
PGO wave is normally observed exclusively in REMS
and in SWS during roughly one minute prior to the
onset of tonic features of REM episodes. However,
in the cat REMS PGO waves are observed during
waking after depletion of brain serotonin (5HT) by
either pharmacological or surgical methods. Initially the emergence of REMS PGO into waking is associated with suppression of sleep, that is, insomnia
(Delorme et al., 1966; Koella et al., 1968). With
chronic 5HT depletion both SWS and REMS periods reappear after about 5 days, but PGO waves continue
to occur during waking as well as during SWS and
REM (Dement et al., 1972). Dement and his
colleagues have suggested that this dissociation
phenomenon may also apply to the dream activity
that is associated with REM in humans. Cats with
waking PGO waves sometimes exhibited components of
"hallucinatory" behaviors simultaneously with the
occurrence of waking PGO bursts. Their behavior
usually consisted of quick jerks of the head and
searching movements, although no external stimuli
were present. Thus, hallucinations may be dreams
occurring in waking. Dement has suggested the PGO

is only one ingredient in the production of hallucinations. However, carcinoid patients, given
tryptophan hydroxylase inhibitors to control a high
level of peripheral serotonin produced by some
tumors, developed florid psychotic hallucinations
which may necessitate discontinuation of treatment
(Engelman et al., 1967).

5. <u>REMS</u> and <u>Waking Without EEG Activation</u>. The
low amplitude "activated" EEG that normally accompanied both waking and REMS, as defined by motor
behavior, may be dissociated from these states
following large focal lesions of the nervous system.
For example, after complete ablation of the thalamus
in cats, the cortical EEG remained synchronized
during episodes of atonia which were accompanied
by pontine spikes, as are normally observed in REMS,
and during behavioral arousal (Villablanca and
Salinas-Zeballo, 1972). As shown in Fig. 10 large
posterior hypothalamus lesions in the rat were also
followed by typical episodes of atonia and behavioral arousal in the absence of EEG change (McGinty,
1969). In both instances the normal EEG-behavioral
associations gradually reappered, after 3 to 5 days
in the rat, and 10 to 25 days in the cat. Interest-
ingly, in both cases, during the course of recovery
from lesions, EEG activation occurred sooner during
REMS than W. As noted above EEG activation also
occurred in AS before W during ontogenetic development.

6. <u>Automatic Behavior Syndromes During Waking</u>.
Certain sleep disorders, including the narcolepsy-
cataplexy syndrome and the sleep-apnea syndrome
are associated with chronic compelling daytime
sleepiness. Most victims of these disorders are
characterized by episodes of inappropriate behavior
denoted as automatic behavior by Guilleminault et
al. (1975). Many individuals report strange dri-
ving incidents including finding that they have
arrived at inappropriate locations while having
amnesia for the intervening time. Traffic accidents
have also occurred. Work and home incidents such
as ripping up important papers, throwing food away,
or putting the dishes in the clothes dryer are also
reported. Apparently routine behaviors may be
continued, but many mistakes occur. Conversations
may take place, but patients may also emit a burst
of words without meaning and without relation to
the ongoing conversation.

In laboratory studies, victims of these

disorders exhibit intermittent deterioration of performance which has been related to the intrusion of sleep-like EEG patterns during ongoing waking behavior (Guilleminault et al., 1975). Patients were asked to carry out routine tasks such as the Wilkinson Addition Test, the Light Stimulus Vigilance Test, or a Serial Alteration Test while EEG activity was monitored continuously. In contrast to control subjects, patients performance would deteriorate after a few minutes. The number of errors would increase, problems were repeated or skipped. These lapses in performance were associated with the intrusion of bursts of stage I EEG or synchronous theta rhythm which are called "micro-sleeps." During these episodes the subjects were frequently seen to stare straight ahead with a blank look.

Many additional examples of waking behavior in the presence of neocortical slow wave activity have been described. This type of phenomenon has been produced by administration of atropine or other anticholinergic drugs in experimental animals, lesions of the thalamus or hypothalamus, and in epileptic patients (see Mirsky and Pragay, 1967 for review). In all of these cases the waking behavior occurring during slow EEG activity is not normal.

7. Waking EEG Patterns During Sleep. Observed EEG patterns during sleep in humans do not always fit the categories provided by widely used scoring manual of Rechtschaffen and Kales (1968). The alpha rhythm is normally associated with a relaxed waking EEG, and may also appear episodically in REMS. Hauri and Hawkins (1973) reported a pattern characterized by alpha-like rhythm (7-10 Hz) associated with 5 to 20% delta waves (0-3 Hz) which seemed to occur instead of stages III and IV. This pattern has been seen in a heterogenious population including patients identified as depressed, schizophrenic, schizoaffective, insomniac, chronically fatigued, temporal lobe epileptic and in a morphine addict, as well as normal 2 to 5 year old children. Hauri and Hawkins noted that many of their adult cases had seen frequent changes in diagnosis during the course of their clinical history and were "diagnostic puzzles." Since this type of state disorganization is associated with a heterogenious

population, a specific physiological interpretation
is difficult to establish, except that mental status
is abnormal or immature.

These studies suggest that the physiological
mechanisms controlling production of either slow
wave EEG activity or activated EEG activity,
suppression of motor behavior, atonia of REMS, PGO
waves of REMS, and the tonic episodes of REMS are
also potentially independent processes that are
normally entrained by the conditions we label as
states. Similar dissociations may apply to particular components of the EEG, and as the alpha rhythm.
However, each of these dissociations is accompanied
by a deviation from optimal behavioral function as
recognized by laboratory tests. These observations
suggest that optimal behavioral function depends
on appropriate state organization. In several
instances the abnormal patterns in adults is found
normally in infants or children. Disorganization
of adult states follows structural lines that are
noted during ontogenetic development of coherent
state patterns. Abnormal infants also exhibit an
absence of well-organized states and state cycling
(Monod et al., 1967; Prechtl et al., 1973). Indeed,
lack of state organization in infants has been
suggested as a sensitive marker of neurological
disturbance.

SUMMARY

Normal mature sleep states are characterized
by the occurrence of specific modes of function
in the autonomic, motor, and EEG systems that are
typically monitored in laboratory studies. Other
studies have revealed state-related manifestations
in many aspects of central nervous system function,
as measured by neuronal unit activity, modulation
of evoked potentials, cerebral blood flow and
metabolism and neuroendocrine function. (For
reviews see Jouvet, 1967; McGinty and Siegel, 1968;
Weitzman, 1976; Steriade and Hobson, 1976; Karnovsky
and Reich, 1977). The studies summarized above
show that the mature organizational features of
sleep state develop gradually, and state organization progresses from an undifferentiated pattern
to gradually more organized, more sustained, states.
AS sleep is most like the primitive state. The
development of mature states appears to have

survival value as shown by studies of resistance of hypoxia.

States may be dissociated in adults. Dissociated states characterize certain clinical populations (narcoleptics, sleep-walkers, hypersomniacs with sleep apnea) as well as influences of central nervous lesions in experimental animals (REM without atonia). Psychiatric populations exhibit disordered and variable temporal patterns in sleep states, see Snyder (1972). All of these observations suggest that optimum behavioral performance is related to organization of sleep states. In other words, sleep has a <u>function</u> in the maintenance of waking behavior, and that function is related to parameters of sleep state organization. A better understanding of specific relationships between sleep state organization and waking behavior patterns is needed (see McGinty and Siegel, 1978). It is likely that this relationship is under selective pressure during evolution.

REFERENCES

Astic, L., and Jouvet-Mounier, D. Mise en evidence du sommeil paradoxal in utero chez le cobaye. <u>Comptes Rendus de la Academie de Sciences</u> (Paris), <u>269</u>: 2578-2581, 1969.

Baker, T. L., and McGinty, D. J. Reversal of cardiopulmonary failure during active sleep in hypoxic kittens: Implications for sudden infant death. <u>Science</u>, <u>198</u>: 419-421, 1977.

Bergman, A. B. Sudden infant death syndrome in King County, Washington. In A. B. Bergman, J. B. Beckwith, and C. G. Ray (Eds.), <u>Sudden Infant Death Syndrome</u>. University of Washington Press, 1970.

Cadilhac, J., Passouant-Fontaine, T., and Passouant, P. L'organisation des divers stades du sommeil chez le chaton, de la naissance a 45 jours. <u>Journal de Physiologie</u>, (Paris), <u>54</u>: 305-306, 1962.

Cadilhac, J., Billiard, M., Halasz, P., and Passouant, P. Les phases transitionnelles du sommeil dans la narcolepsie et l'epilepsie. Revue de Electroencephalographie et de Neurophysiologie. 3: 153-164, 1973.

Chase, M. H. Brain stem somatic reflex activity in neonatal kittens during sleep and wakefulness. Physiology and Behavior, 1: 165-172, 1971.

Chase, M. H., McGinty, D. J., and Sterman, M. B. Cyclic variation in the amplitude of a brain stem reflex during sleep and wakefulness. Experientia, 24: 47, 1968.

Coccagna, G., Mantovani, M., Brignani, F., Parchi, C., and Lugaresi, E. Continous recording of the pulmonary and systemic arterial pressure during sleep in syndromes of hypersomnia with periodic breathing. Bulletin of Physiopathology, 8: 1159-1172, 1972.

Delange, M., Caston, P., Cadilhac, J., and Passouant, P. Les divers studes du sommeil chez le nouveau-ne et nourrison. Revue de Neurologie, 107: 271-276, 1962.

Delorme, F., Froment, J. L., Jouvet, M. Suppression du sommeil par la P-chloremathamphetamine et de la P-chlorophenylalanine. Comptes Rendus de la Societe de Biologie, 160: 2347-2351, 1966.

Dement, W., Rechtschaffen, A., and Gulevitch, G. The mature of the narcoleptic sleep attack. Neurology, 16: 18-33, 1966.

Dement, W. C., Mitler, M. M., and Henriksen, S. J. Sleep changes during chronic administration of parachlorophenylalanine. Revue Canadienne de Biologie, 31 (suppl): 239-246, 1972.

Dreyfus-Brisac, C. Sleep ontogenesis in early human prematurity from 24 to 27 weeks of conceptual age. Developmental Psychobiology, 1: 162-169, 1968.

Engelman, K., Lovenberg, W., and Sjoerdsma, A.
    Inhibition of serotonin synthesis by para-
    chlorophenylalanine in patients with the
    carcinoid syndrome. New England Journal of
    Medicine, 277: 1103-1108, 1967.

Foix, C. Maladie de Parkinson, Lesions. Revue
    de Neurologie, 7: 593-630, 1921.

Gastaut, H., Tassinari, C. A., and Duron, B. Poly-
    graphic study of the episodic diurnal and
    nocturnal (hypnic and respiratory) manifesta-
    tions of the Pickwick syndrome. Brain Research,
    2: 167-186, 1966.

Glotzbach, S. F., and Heller, H. B. Central
    nervous regulation of body temperature during
    sleep. Science, 194: 537-539, 1976.

Guilleminault, C., Phillips, R., and Dement, W. C.
    A syndrome of hypersomnia with automatic
    behavior. Electroencephalography and Clinical
    Neurophysiology, 38(4): 403-413, 1975.

Hauri, P. and Hawkinds, D. R. Alpha-delta sleep.
    Electroencephalography and Clinical Neuro-
    physiology, 34: 233-237, 1973.

Helbrügge, T. The development of circadian rhythms
    in infants. Cold Springs Harbor Symposia on
    Quantitative Biology, 25: 311-323, 1960.

Henley, K., and Morrison, A. R. A re-evaluation
    of the effects of lesions of the pontine
    tegmentum and locus coeruleus on phenomena of
    paradoxical sleep in the cat. Acta Neuro-
    biologia Experimentale, 34: 215-232, 1974.

Hoppenbrouwers, T. and Sterman, M. B. Development
    of sleep state patterns in the kitten.
    Experimental Neurology, 49: 822-838, 1975.

Iwamura, Y., Tsuda, K., Kudo, N., and Kohana, K.
    Monosynaptic reflex during natural sleep in
    the kitten. Brain Research, 11: 456-459, 1968.

Jacobson, A., Kales, A., Lehmann, D., and Zweig, J.
    R. Somnambulism: All-night electroencephalo-
    graphic studies. Science, 148: 975-977, 1965.

Jeannerod, M., and Sakai, K.   Occipital and genicu-
    late potentials related to eye movement in
    the unanesthetized cat.   Brain Research, 19:
    361-377, 1970.

Jones, B. E., Harper, S. T., and Halaris, A. E.
    Effects of locus coeruleus lesions upon
    cerebral monoamine content, sleep wakefulness
    states, and response to amphetamine in the
    cat.   Brain Research, 124: 473-496, 1977.

Jouvet, M.   Recherches sur les structures nerveuses
    et les mecanisme responsables des differentes
    phases du sommeil physiologique.   Archives
    Italiannes de Biologie, 100: 125-206, 1962.

Jouvet, M.   Neurophysiology of the states of sleep.
    Physiology Reviews, 42: 117-177, 1967.

Jouvet-Mounier, D., Astic, L., and Lacote, D.
    Ontogenesis of the states of sleep in rat,
    cat, and guinea pig during the first postnatal
    month.   Developmental Psychobiology, 2: 216-
    239, 1970.

Karnovsky, M. L., and Reich, P.   Biochemistry of
    sleep.   In B. W. Agronoff and M. H. Aprison
    (Eds.), Advances in Neurochemistry, Vol.2,
    Plenum, 1977, pp. 213-275.

Koella, W. P., Feldstein, A., and Czicman, J. S.
    The effect of para-chloro-phenylalanine on
    the sleep of cats.   Electroencephalogrphy
    and Clinical Neurophysiology, 25: 481-490,
    1968.

MacGregor, M. C., Block, A. J., and Ball, W. C. Jr.
    Topics in clinical medicine serious complica-
    tions and sudden death in the Pickwickian
    syndrome.   Johns Hopkins Medical Journal, 126:
    279-295, May 1970.

McGinty, D. J.   Somnolence, recovery, and hyposomnia
    following ventro-medial diencephalic lesions
    in the rat.   Electroencephalography and
    Clinical Neurophysiology, 26: 70-79, 1969.

McGinty, D. J. Encephalization and the neural
    control of sleep. In M. B. Sterman, D. J.
    McGinty and A. M. Adinolfi (Eds.), Brain
    Development and Behavior. Academic Press,
    New York, 1971, pp. 335-357.

McGinty, D. J., Stevenson, M., Hoppenbrouwers, T.,
    Harper, R. M., Sterman, M. B., and Hodgman, J.
    Polygraphic studies of kitten development:
    Sleep state patterns. Developmental Psycho-
    biology, 10: 455-469, 1977.

McGinty, D. J., and Siegel, J. M. Sleep states.
    In E. Satinoff and P. Teitelbaum (Eds.).
    Motivation. Handbook of Neurobiology, 1978,
    in press.

Mirsky, A. F., and Pragay, E. B. The relation of
    EEG and performance in altered states of
    consciousness. In S. S. Kety, E. V. Evarts,
    and H. L. Williams (Eds.), Sleep and Altered
    States of Consciousness. Vol. 45. Baltimore:
    Williams and Wilkinson Co., 1967, pp. 514-534.

Monod, N., Dreyfus-Brisac, C., Morel-Kahn, S.,
    Pajot, N., and Plassard, N. Les premieres
    etapes de l'organisation du sommeil chez le
    premature et le nouveau-ne. Revue de Neuro-
    logie, 110: 304-305, 1964.

Monod, N., Eliet-Flescher, J., and Dreyfus-Brisac,
    C. Le sommeil du nouveau-ne et du premature.
    III. Les troubles de l'organization du sommeil
    chez le nouveau-ne pathologique. Biologie
    Neonatale, 11: 216-247, 1967.

Mouret, J. Differences in sleep in patients with
    Parkinson's disease. Electroencephalography
    and Clinical Neurophysiology, 38: 653-657, 1975.

Naeye, R. L. Pulmonary arterial abnormalities in
    the sudden death syndrome. New England Journal
    of Medicine, 289: 1167-1170, 1973.

Naeye, R. L. Hypoxemia and the sudden infant death
    syndrome. Science, 186: 837-838, 1974.

Parmeggiani, P. L. and Rabini, C.   Sleep and environmental temperature.   Archives Italiannes
de Biologie, 108: 369-387, 1970.

Parmeggiani, P. L., and Sabattini, L.   Electromyographic aspects of postural, respiratory
and thermoregulatory mechanisms in sleeping
cats.   Electroencephalography and Clinical
Neurophysiology, 33: 1-13, 1972.

Parmelee, A. H. and Stern, E.   Development of states
in infants.   In C. D. Clemente, D. P. Purpura,
and F. E. Mayer (Eds.), Sleep and the Maturing
Nervous System.   New York: Academic Press,
1972, pp. 199-215.

Parmelee, A. H., Wenner, W. H., Akiyama, Y.,
Schultz, M., and Stern, E.   Sleep states in
premature infants.   Developmental Medicine and
Child Neurology, 9: 70-77, 1967.

Phillipson, E., and Sullivan, C.   Respiratory
control mechanisms during non-REM and REM
sleep.   In C. Ghilleminault and W. C. Dement
(Eds.), Sleep Apnea Syndromes.   New York:
Alan R. Liss, Inc., 1978, in press.

Pompeiano, O.   The neurophysiological mechanisms
of the postural and motor events during
desynchronized sleep.   In S. S. Kety, E. V.
Evarts, and H. L. Williams (Eds.), Sleep and
Altered States of Consciousness. Research
Publication of the Association of Nervous
Mental Diseases, vol. 45, 1967, pp. 351-423.

Prechtl, H. F. R., Theorell, K. and Blair, A. W.
Behavioral states cycles in abnormal infants.
Developmental Medicine and Child Neurology,
15: 606-615, 1973.

Rechtschaffen, A., Wolpert, E., Dement, W.,
Mitchaell, S., and Fisher, C.   Nocturnal
sleep of narcoleptics.   Electroencephalography
and Clinical Neurophysiology, 15: 599-609,
1963.

Rechtschaffen, A. and Kales, A. A Manual of Standardized Terminology, Techniques and Scoring System for Sleep Stages of Human Subjects. Public Health Service, U. S. Printing Office, 1968.

Roffwarg, H. P., Muzio, J. N. and Dement, W. C. Ontogenetic development of the human sleep-dream cycle. Science, 152: 604-619, 1966.

Snyder, F. Electroencephalographic studies of sleep in psychiatric disorders. In. M. H. Chase (Ed.), The Sleeping Brain. Brain Information Service, Los Angeles, 1972, pp. 376-393.

Steinschneider, A. Prolonged apnea and the sudden infant death syndrome: Clinical and laboratory observations. Pediatrics, 50: 646-654, 1972.

Steriade, M. and Hobson, J. A. Neuronal activity during the sleep-waking cycle. Progress in Neurobiology, 6: 155-376, 1976.

Steriade, M., Deschenes, M., and Oakson, G. Inhibitory processes and interneuronal apparatus in motor cortex during sleep and waking. I. Background firing and responsiveness of pyramidal tract neurons and interneurons. Journal of Neurophysiology, 73: 1065-1092, 1974.

Stevenson, M., and McGinty, D. J. Polygraphic studies of kitten development: Respiratory rate and variability. Developmental Psychobiology, 1978, in press.

Villablanca, J. and Salinas-Zeballos, M. E. Sleep-wakefulness, EEG and behavioral studies of chronic cats without the thalamus - the "athalamic cat". Archives Italiannes de Biologie, 110, 383-411, 1972.

Weitzman, E. D. Circadian rhythms and episodic hormone secretion in man. Annual Review of Medicine, 27: 225-243, 1976.

Wellens, H. J. J., Vermeulen, A., and Durrer, D.
    Ventricular fibrillation occurring on arousal
    from sleep by auditory stimuli. Circulation,
    46: 661-665, 1972.

Yoss, R. E., Daly, D. D. Criteria for the diagnosis
    of the narcoleptic syndrome. Proceedings
    of the Mayo Clinic, 32: 320-328, 1957.

ONTOGENY OF SLEEP: IMPLICATIONS FOR FUNCTION

M. B. STERMAN

V. A. Hospital, Sepulveda, California
and
UCLA School of Medicine, Los Angeles, California

Everybody knows what sleep is for. We all use it every day. We use it when we can no longer function adequately while awake, we use it in preparation for a busy day ahead, we use it when we are bored and when we wish to turn off the unacceptable circumstances of adversity. Yet these obvious human experiences with sleep do not define a function which is comprehensible from a mechanistic point of view. Certainly sleep must have some fundamental role in biological economy, but both the complexity of this process as we now know it and the diversity of neural organization across phylogeny contribute to a continuing debate, as evidenced by this text. In addressing this problem over the years, while at the same time attempting to comprehend developmental data being generated in our laboratory, I have become convinced that the functions of sleep cannot be adequately examined unless the multiple physiological components of this process are properly sorted out. The study of sleep from a developmental perspective provides for a natural dissection, since these components appear to emerge in a systematic manner.

If one examines long-term polygraphic data from a very young infant, a single, dominant characteristic emerges. That characteristic is periodicity. The most prominent periodicity observed is an alternation of physiological patterns describing a cycle of approximately 60 minutes. Figure 1 shows integrated polygraphic data from a continuous 12 hour recording period in a 30 day old infant. It can be seen that EEG, autonomic and somatic measures are all organized in a very basic sense by this cycle. The classification of states has become a fundamental tool in sleep research and, from that point of view this cycle is attributed to the alternation of REM and non-REM states across the night. However, Kleitman

Copyright © 1979 by Academic Press, Inc.
All rights of reproduction in any form reserved.
ISBN 0-12-222340-3

(1963) suggested that this periodicity in the
infant reflected a "basic rest-activity cycle" or
BRAC, which he equated to primitive sleep and
waking states. He viewed these states as precursors
to more advanced states of sleep and wakefulness
which would emerge subsequent to central nervous
system maturation. As can be seen in Figure 1,
the non-REM phase of this cycle is characterized
by high voltage EEG activity, a decrease in cardiac
and respiratory rate and variability, and a relative absence of phasic movements. In fact, the
attenuation of visceral and somatic activities seen
in this state produces the lowest levels of function registered throughout the 24 hour day. Empirically, then, the non-REM state is truly a rest
period, in the usual sense of that term.

Developmental research has addressed the
questions of the origin and neural substrates for
this organization. Studies in our laboratory some
years ago suggested that the human fetus possessed
a 40-60 minute periodicity in somatic activity
detectable as early as 24 weeks gestational age
(Sterman, 1967; Sterman and Hoppenbrouwers, 1971).
In recent years unequivocal evidence for the
occurrence of this cycle in lower animals has
accumulated. Astic and Jouvet-Mounier (1969)
collected polygraphic data showing recurrent REM
states in the fetal guinea pig. Extensive data
of this kind were reported also in the fetal lamb
(Ruckebusch, 1972; Maloney, 1977) and monkey
(Martin et al., 1974). More recently, noninvasive
measures of heart rate and respiratory movements
in the human fetus have supported the existence
of a physiological periodicity approximating 40-50
minutes (Sterman et al., 1973; Hoppenbrouwers
et al., 1977; Patrick, 1977). It seems apparent,
then, that the REM-nonREM or BRAC organization of
states arises in prenatal neural development.

Total removal of the forebrain in the cat
does not abolish this cycle. Jouvet (1962, 1967)
was the first to demonstrate this fact, and to
show that the primary behavior remaining in such
a preparation was a continuous alternation of
tonic and atonic states closely resembling the
pattern of REM-nonREM states seen in the intact
animal (Figure 2). He concluded from these studies
that the sleep mechanism was localized to structures
in the pontine brain stem.

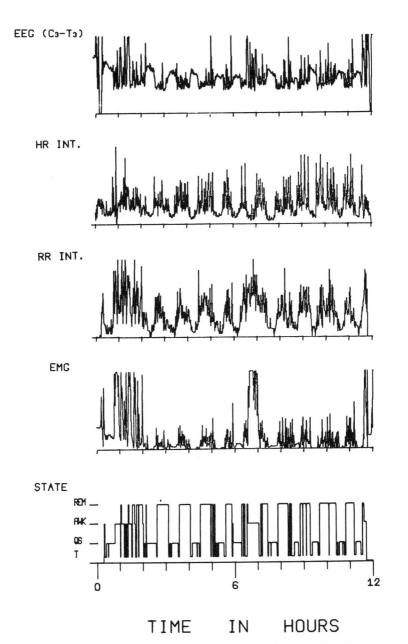

EEG (C₃–T₃)

HR INT.

RR INT.

EMG

STATE

REM —
AWK —
QS —
T

0   6   12

TIME   IN   HOURS

Fig. 1 The importance of basic periodicity
in polygraphic measurements from infants can best
be appreciated if long-term recordings are obtained
and plotted in a compressed format such as shown

These facts raise some important questions.
Can the process that "ravels up the tattered sleeve
of care" reside solely within brain stem structures
or serve a purpose in the fetus and newborn similar
to its complex manifestations in adults? Certainly
the fetus and newborn have no waking function to
sustain, nor do they anticipate or avoid the coming
day. It is possible, however, that they are bored.
Nevertheless, parsimony demands that the periodicity in fetus and newborn physiology be considered a more primitive manifestation of state organization in mammals, as suggested by Kleitman's
BRAC. We have reviewed the evidence in favor of
this conclusion in several previous reports
(Sterman and Hoppenbrouwers, 1971; Sterman, 1972).
Some have argued against the concept of a
basic rest-activity cycle on the grounds that the
REM cycle does not obey the principles of an intrinsic biological clock. It is unlikely that
Kleitman intended such an interpretation, and
certainly those investigators who have examined
this concept in terms of a modulating influence
in wakefulness have never found evidence for an
internal clock. What has been demonstrated in
several mammals is an ultradian periodicity in a
number of behaviors and functions, the major
characteristic of which is a period and variability

Fig. 1 continued:

here. These data were recorded continuously over
a 12 hour period (8 PM - 8 AM) from a 30-day-old
infant. Left central cortical EEG voltage and
chin muscle EMG voltage were integrated on a
minute-by-minute basis, while cardiac beat-to-beat
intervals (HR INT) and respiratory breath-to-breath
intervals (RR INT) were summarized as minute-by-
minute medians. A corresponding visual state classification across the night is shown also. The
spontaneous modulation of these variables describes
a cycle of approximately 60 minutes. The quiet
state was characterized by high voltage EEG
patterns, low and stable cardiac and respiratory
cycles and a low level of muscle activity. Conversely, both REM and awake (AWK) states showed
increased and irregular visceral and somatic
activities and a low voltage EEG pattern.

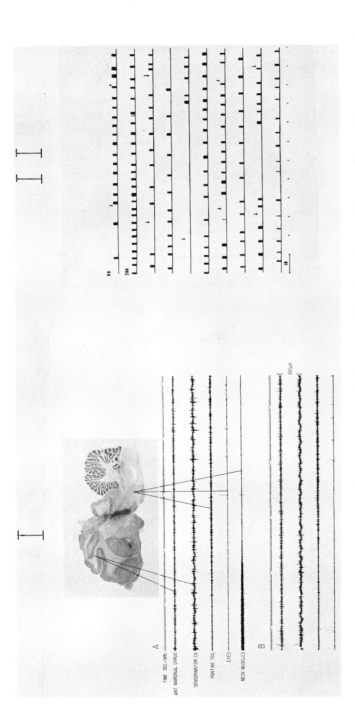

Fig. 2. Evidence for a basic rest-activity cycle is shown here from two separate experiments which employed surgical transection of the neuraxis in the cat. Data shown at I are from Sterman (1974), and depict the independent occurrence of a brain stem REM cycle and a cortical EEG sleep-wake cycle in a cat with brain transected at caudal diencephalon. Data at II are from Jouvet (1965), and who recurrence of REM periods in a surviving pontine cat over a five day period of continous monitoring. Time, in hours, is shown at bottom at lines show REM episodes (black rectangles) over successive 12 hour periods of recording. Arrows indicate times of exaphageal intubation for feeding.

similar to that of the REM cycle (Othmer et al.,
1969; Globus, 1970; Sterman et al., 1972; Kripke,
1974). For our own part, we have proposed that
the periodicity results from certain temporal
characteristics of cellular metabolism which are
sensed by brain stem mechanisms capable of adjust-
ing integrated function appropriately. Thus, the
observed periodicity can be compared to other
periodic regulatory functions, such as breathing
or swallowing. These behaviors also have substrates organized in the brain stem. Periodicity
in their expression results from interactions related to the increase and decrease of complex
physiological and biochemical stimuli impinging
upon reflex pathways. These stimuli, in turn, are
modulated by other influences which determine
their intensity and distribution in time. In the
mature system, the entire mechanism can be brought
under the partial control of forebrain functions
which can disrupt periodicity or readily alter the
phase characteristics of the cycle. Such may be
the case also with the REM cycle; however, the
specific stimuli and brain stem substrates involved
remain unclear at the present time.

In summary, it is proposed once again that
early state organization in the human infant is
dominated by a 40-60 minute basic-rest-activity
cycle which is an intrinsic brain stem regulatory
function. This cycle makes its initial appearance
in fetal development as the substrates for basic
physiological regulation become functional. The
existence of this periodicity is seen as an evolutionary endowment which provides the newborn with
an efficient state organization as it begins the
complex process of post-natal development.

Several major changes characterize the development of state organization after birth. Periods of generalized arousal, which originally occurred briefly at 3-4 hour intervals, lengthen dramatically (Parmelee et al., 1964) as motor and social learning during these periods give rise to the state of wakefulness. Periods of quiescence within the rest-activity cycle also lengthen significantly, and become associated with specific EEG patterns characteristic of adult quiet sleep (Parmelee and Stern, 1972; Sterman et al., 1977). Finally this quiescence, still modulated by relatively unchanged periods of nonspecific activation (REM), shifts progressively into the nocturnal phase of the circadian cycle (Figure 3). As with phylogeny, forebrain maturation in ontogeny provides for a more advanced state organization, characterized by a circadian sleep-waking cycle superimposed on an ultradian rest-activity cycle, the expression of which is still apparent during sleep. This interpretation is only slightly different from the position taken by Kleitman (1963) on the basis primarily, of intuition. It is also consistent to some extent with the distinction made earlier by Jouvet (1960) between slow wave or non-REM sleep, which he attributed to forebrain organization and termed "telencephalic sleep," and REM sleep, which he felt was organized in the brain stem and dubbed as "rhombencephalic sleep."

Thus, while the rest activity cycle may be considered as a "pre-wired" function of the brain stem, perhaps a product of evolutionary forces seeking an efficient system for energy conservation, sleep and wakefulness arise with forebrain maturation and are products of the complex interaction of nature and nurture. Viewed in this way the development of sleep is a post-natal phenomenon, subject both to the dictates of physiological maturation and the influences of environment. Such factors as geography and social custom entrain the physiological substrates of the sleep-waking cycle and determine the behavioral patterns which will come to characterize these states in a given culture.

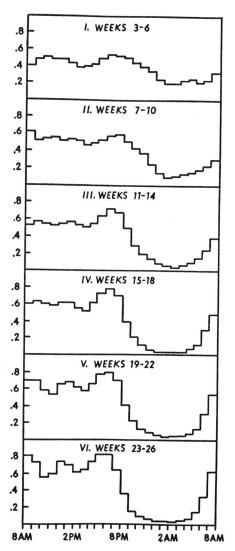

Fig. 3. Twenty-four distribution of observed
waking activity in a group of infants tabulated
across six successive four-week periods in early
development. Mean proportion of wakefulness
(ordinate) is plotted against clock time (abscissa).
Sleep periods are indicated as reciprocal of waking.
Note that circadian modulation is essentially absent
to six weeks of life and well developed by 11-14
weeks (from Kleitman and Engelmann, 1953).

We have had the opportunity recently to carefully evaluate some of the dictates of physiological
maturation in local infants through extensive polygraphic studies of the development of sleep. At
the time of this writing, data from ten neurologic-
ally normal infants of gestational ages between
39-41 weeks have been sufficiently analyzed for
consideration in this context. Birth weights in
these infants ranged between 3000-4000 grams, and
all were full term and appropriate for gestational
age according to standard intrauterine growth
curves (Usher and McLean, 1969). Each infant was
monitored polygraphically during continous 12 hour
sessions at one week of age and at monthly intervals
to six months of age. Each recording session began
at approximately 8 P.M.

Some description of the recording situation
will be useful in interpreting our results. Monitoring was carried out in a darkened recording room
kept at 23-25 degrees centigrade. Infants were fed
during application of electrodes, and newborns were
swaddled prior to the initiation of recording. Arm
restraints were applied to older infants in order
to prevent disruption of electrodes. EEG recordings
were obtained bilaterally with electrode placements
approximating T_3-C_3 and T_4-C_4, according to the
international 10-20 system. To provide for sleep
stage scoring chin EMG and eye movements were
recorded also. Respiration was monitored by thoracic
impedance, a nasal thermistor, and end expired pCO_2
measurements, using a Beck LB-2 CO_2 monitor. ECG
was measured through two disposable electrodes
placed symmetrically beneath the clavicles, with a
ground electrode applied above the umbilicus. Finally, gross somatic activity was recorded through
Mylar-coated conductive sensors positioned under
the crib mattress.

Data were recorded on a 16-channel analog
tape, together with an IRIG E time code. All recording instruments were in an adjacent room, and
their operation in no way disrupted the sleeping
infant. Behavior was also monitored continuously
with the use of a low illumination video camera
and monitor. Events such as closing and opening
of eyes, startle, crying and vocalization, as well
as nursing interventions were charted at the
appropriate time on the polygraphic record.

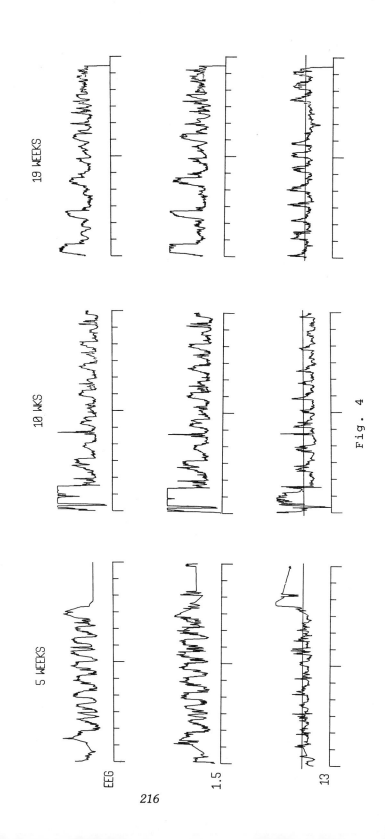

Fig. 4

Fig. 4. Integrated EEG data from left central cortex (C_3-T_3) is shown here as obtained from an infant during continuous 12 hour recordings at 5, 10 and 19 weeks of age. The abscissa for all plots shows time in hours from 8 PM-8 AM. Top plots at all ages (EEG) show minute-by-minute integrated total voltage as in figure 1. Other plots show minute integrated voltage after band-pass filtering of the EEG signal through filters detecting 3 Hz bands centered at 1.5 and 13 Hz, respectively. Note that at 5 weeks the modulation of total EEG power is determined by activity in the 0-3 Hz band almost exclusively. By 10 weeks of age a corresponding periodicity in 12-14 Hz activity becomes apparent. At 19 weeks activity in the two bands tends to separate, with 12-15 Hz modulation now reflecting the rest-activity cycle and 0-3 Hz activity becoming organized according to a slower periodicity. This shift appears to reflect the emergence of a mature sleep-waking process between 10-20 weeks of age, as in figure 3.

217

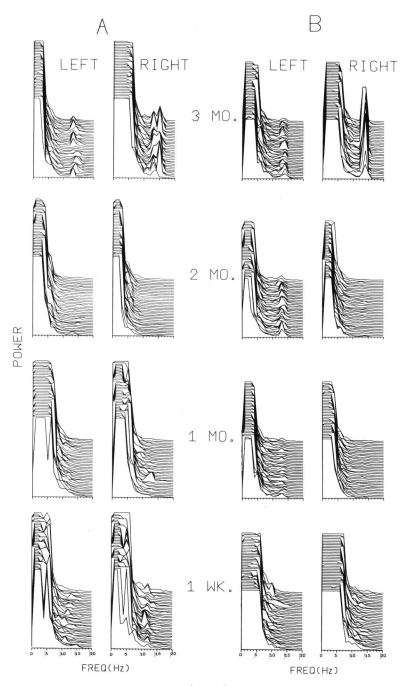

Fig. 5

Polygraphic variables recorded on analog tape were pre-treated and processed with a PDP-12 computer. The analysis of each variable involved complex computer applications, all of which have been described in detail elsewhere (Harper et al., 1976; Hoppenbrouwers et al., 1977; Sterman et al., 1977). While these and other analytic procedures have been applied to all data recorded throughout the night, the present discussion will focus on the quiet phase of the rest-activity cycle, since developmental changes are most dramatic for this state.

Fig. 5. Isometric power-spectral plots are shown here for 10 minutes samples of quiet sleep taken from the middle of the night in two infants. Left and right central cortical plots are from data sampled between 1 and 12 weeks of age. Traces were derived from successive 16 second epochs of EEG data. The amplitude of low frequencies was limited in these plots in order to scale for resolution of higher frequencies. Data from infant A shows characteristic pattern, with some spindle frequency activity (12-15 Hz) apparent at one week of age, but little detected at 4 and 8 weeks. At 12 weeks of age well developed spindle frequencies are seen bilaterally. Data from infant B show similar pattern over right central cortex, but less common progressive development of spindles on the left side (from Sterman et al., 1977).

Despite its well elaborated shortcomings, the EEG provides one of the best, noninvasive indices of central nervous system development available at the present time. In our studies, this parameter was evaluated quantitatively through both bandpass and power-spectral analysis. For bandpass analysis EEG signals were subjected to electronic bandpass pre-filtering and plotted as integrated activity for selected frequency bands on a minute-by-minute basis, over the 12 hour recording period. This analysis provided an interesting perspective on develpmental periodicities as reflected by voltage-frequency components of the EEG. Figure 4 shows a typical developmental progression, with integrated total EEG voltage, integrated voltage in a three Hz frequency band centered at 1.5 Hz and integrated relative power in a three Hz band centered at 13 Hz, all expressed over 12 hours of recording time. At five weeks of age there is a strong reflection of the rest-activity cycle in total EEG voltage, which results primarily from modulation of low frequency activity. The period of this cycle is approximately 60 minutes. By 10 weeks a significant 12-14 Hz component is apparent in the EEG. This component is modulated concurrently with low fre-quency patterns during the rest-activity cycle. The low frequency component appears to be somewhat attenuated during alternate cycles at this age. When the infant has reached 19 weeks of age (almost five months) a new organization has emerged. The rest-activity cycle continues to be manifest as a periodicity of approximately 60 minutes; however, this cycle is now reflected primarily by modulation of 12-14 Hz activity. Periodicity in the 1-3 Hz band has lengthened, in this case to manifest a coupled cycle of about two hours.

A different perspective of these changes can be provided by a review of findings using yet another method of quantitative analysis. The recorded EEG signals were also digitized and analyzed with Fast

Fourier transform. Sequential spectra from 16 second samples were adjusted by reference to a calibration spectral peak and plotted isometrically to provide compressed spectral arrays depicting the distribution of power across time (Fig. 5). Spectral valued from selected samples were subjected to log transformation and sorted into five 4 Hz bands between 0-19 Hz, corresponding partially to the designation by Davis et al. (1938) of delta (0-3 Hz), theta (4-7 Hz), alpha (8-11 Hz), sigma (12-15 Hz) and beta (16-19 Hz) EEG frequencies.

A summary of developmental patterns as reflected by the distribution of central cortical EEG spectral densities during QS is shown in Figure 6. Asterisks in this figure denote statistically significant changes with age. It can be seen that the activity in the 0-3 Hz frequency band increased progressively during the first two months of life, while all other frequencies tended to be diminished. Activity in the 12-15 Hz band was actually reduced significantly at four weeks, as compared to one and eight weeks of age. Activity at 0-3 Hz remained stable after eight weeks, but 12-15 Hz power increased significantly to twelve weeks. Power in the 4-7 and 8-11 Hz bands did not show significant change until sixteen weeks of age.

The implications of these findings are best appreciated from an anatomical point of view. Early forebrain maturation proceeds according to a systematic schedule. As far as EEG substrates are concerned, the earliest elements to mature appear to be the apical dendrites of cortical pyramidal cells (Scheibel and Scheibel, 1964). These elements provide the substrate for receptive interaction among cortical cells and it is their synchronous activity which is thought to produce diffuse slow waves in the EEG. Thus, the early developmental increment in delta activity could be viewed as an indication of an emerging intracortical communication which takes precedence over other connectivity at this stage of development. Overlapping with this phase, but somewhat delayed, are the maturation of dendritic spines and basilar dendritic structures (Scheibel and Scheibel, 1971). These elements receive afferent sensory information and are involved in the intricate patterns of thalamo-cortical interactions which provide the substrate for rhythmic activity in the EEG. This fact may

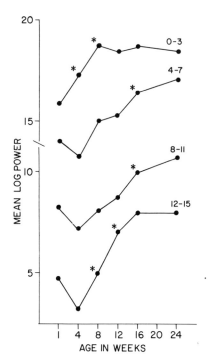

Fig. 6. Developmental changes in the distribution of EEG power during quiet state in a group
of eight normal infants. Four successive 4 Hz frequency bands were evaluated through power-spectral
analysis of beginning, middle and end of night
samples of quiet "sleep" state. Asterisks indicate
statistically significant changes from previous
values. Note early increase in low frequency power
associated with a clear decrease in spindle frequencies. This pattern changes after 4 weeks of
age with 12-15 Hz activity showing developmental
reversal towards marked increase at 12 weeks.

account for the delayed appearance of 12-15 Hz sleep
spindles (sigma activity) and other rhythmic frequencies (theta and alpha). The latter frequencies
are more prominent in the waking EEG of older infants and adults. These findings suggest that
thalamocortical communication becomes possible only
after the cortical receptive elements are ready for

signal processing. Likewise, the development of
sleep and waking functions, which depend upon these
same neural elements, await the maturational sequence of essential substrates, a process which
appears to require about three months. During
this hiatus, state organization is accomplished
by basic reflex mechanisms of the brain stem which
have been functional since before birth.

The transition from a fetal-newborn organization to the more mature state organization of the
older infant is itself a complex process. A comparison of the developmental characteristics of
several physiological parameters provides for a
broader perspective of this process than the EEG
alone can afford. Figure 7 shows median heart
rates, respiratory rates and total somatic activity
from samples of the quiet state in healthy infants
during the first six months of life. Shown also
is the re-scaled developmental pattern for 12-15 Hz
central cortical EEG activity from Figure 6. Each
parameter undergoes a somewhat unique developmental
sequence; however, it becomes clear that there are
distinct, overall stages in this sequencing.

The newborn provides a reference point for
comparison. It will be recalled that state organization here is primarily a 40-60 minute periodicity with generalized arousals occurring at
approximately 2-5 hour intervals. Also, the quiet
state at this stage shows the lowest and most
stable levels of visceral and somatic activity.
By four weeks of age many changes have occurred
and a second stage of development becomes apparent.
Heart rate has increased significantly in all
states (Harper et al., 1976), while 12-15 Hz EEG
activity during quiescence has decreased (Sterman
et al., 1977). Both respiratory rate and somatic
activity have begun a steady decline which will
reach statistical significance by 12 weeks of age.
What defines this second stage is the peculiar
reversal in developmental trend seen after four
weeks, with heart rate declining to greatly reduced,
stable levels by 12 weeks and sleep spindle activity emerging clearly in the EEG between 8-12 weeks.

This reversal in developmental trend, centered at approximately four weeks in a number of
measurements, raises some interesting possibilities for interpretation. Why are some neural
functions apparently more mature at birth, in

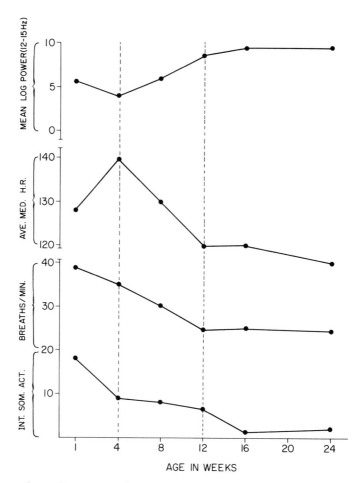

Fig. 7. Developmental changes in mean EEG,
visceral and somatic measures during quiet "sleep"
state in a group of eight normal infants. Values
were derived by combining data from three 10
minute samples obtained at beginning, middle and
end of recording period. Mean log power in the
12-15 Hz band as determined by power-spectral
analysis (figures 5 and 6) is shown at top. Average median heart rate and breaths per minute as
well as mean integrated somatic activity during
these same samples were computed from data such as
that shown in figure 1. A developmental reversal

terms of eventual developmental patterns, than
they are weeks later? During this period adaptive
fetal mechanisms are gradually replaced by developing infant regulatory functions. This switchover,
however, is sometimes buffered by maternal endowment, which results in protection of the highly
vulnerable newborn. For example, the gamma globulin level of the newborn infant is as high as
that of his mother, but decreases rapidly during
the first month after birth, reaching its nadir
then increasing again after three months
(Orlandini et al., 1955). While the fetus manu-
factures its own albumin and alpha and beta glo-
bulins, virtually its entire gamma globulin store
is maternal in origin, acquired by placental transfer. In particular, the gamma-2 fraction, which
is primarily associated with antibody activity,
crosses the placenta readily and makes up the bulk
of the newborn infant's gamma globulin (Schaffer
et al., 1965). Thus maternally acquired antibody
activity is high in the newborn, but is attenuated
by depletion and restored by eventual maturation
of an endogenous source. Similarly, the newborn
infant may possess the capacity for some degree
of mature physiological regulation by virtue of
the availability of essential humoral mediators
acquired through placental transfer. This endowment would buffer the disruptive, disorganizing
influences of parturition and aid the newborn
during its first critical period of extrauterine
existence. During subsequent weeks these mediators
would be depleted, but the impact of this loss
would be countered by rapid post-natal neuronal
maturation and the beginnings of their endogenous
replacement by developing systems in the infant.
These dynamics, whatever their basis, suggest that
physiology is busy with a number of important developmental tasks in addition to neuronal

---

in 12-15 Hz EEG activity and in heart rate is
apparent after 4 weeks of age. The sharp drop in
somatic activity seen between 1-4 weeks is
attenuated thereafter until 16 weeks of age. Respiratory rate showed a steady decline to 12 weeks
of age. All measures became significantly more
stable after the third month of post-natal life.

maturation during the first months of extrauterine
life. Behavioral development during this same
period is sluggish, and state organization remains
basically unchanged, despite important maturational adjustments.

Dramatic changes occur, however, between one
and three months of age, leading to a third stage
in sleep development. This stage is characterized
by greatly reduced levels of somatic and visceral
activity, and an EEG pattern marked by both slow
waves and spindles. Rapid post-natal change has
been replaced by more stable functions which will
continue to approach adult levels at a retarded
pace. At this point in development, circadian
rhythms are well established and sustained waking
increasingly dominated the daylight hours, while a
mature sleep process becomes increasingly concen-
trated during the night. This sleep process is
characterized by prolonged quiet periods, with low
and stable levels of visceral and somatic activities. Numerous studies have shown that at this
age rapid motor and social development begins to
occur. The first steps of a long developmental
journey are over, and, with maturation complete
to the point of a stable sleep-waking organization,
new and complex tasks can now be undertaken.

SUMMARY AND THEORETICAL CONCLUSIONS

The model of the development of sleep proposed
above provides for the mechanistic approach to its
functions sought earlier in this discussion.
Physiology in all of its manifestations requires a
balance between opposing components in the expression of function, a balance which can be identified at each level of organization in the hier-
archy leading to behavior. Thus, in the respiratory system, plasma oxygen vs. carbon dioxide
pressures and acid-base balance determine neural
excitation and inhibition, which in turn produce
specific patterns of muscular contraction and
relaxation giving rise to inspiration and expiration. Basic to all function, however, is the
overall state of the organism, and this parameter
of state must also abide the need for balance.
It is proposed that the ultimate behavioral

consequence of the need for balanced physiological function at all levels is a rest-activity cycle which, in mammals, is organized through the interaction of multiple brain stem regulatory mechanisms. This cycle is an expression of physiology and not its master, and is therefore variable in nature and subject to disruption. Its phylogenetic emergence is recapitulated in ontogeny.

With both evolutionary encephalization and forebrain maturation a new organization is made possible, one which responds to the dictates of a more complex existence. In man and other mammals, the survival value of a prolonged active period creates the requirement of a consolidated state of rest. From this emerges a cycle of wakefulness and sleep which remains coupled to the more primitive rest-activity cycle. Sleep is initiated during a rest phase and terminated with an activity phase. The rest-activity cycle may thus provide a basic unit of physiological time, not a fixed unit, but a unit responsive to internal conditions. In this context, the rest-activity cycle may also provide an important regulatory role during sleep in the mature system. There is evidence that the attenuation of visceral and somatic functions during quiet sleep can, under some circumstances, lead to failure and death unless and active sleep phase is initiated (Baker and McGinty, 1977). Thus, this cycle may also perform an homeostatic function making possible a sustained sleep state during which restorative processes occur in a quantum fashion.

ACKNOWLEDGEMENTS

The research reported here was supported by the Veterans Administration and several federal grants and contracts, in particular NIH NICHD HD4-2810, "Developmental Phenomena and the Occurrence of SIDS." In addition, the author wishes to acknowledge the important contributions to this work by Drs. Toke Hoppenbrouwers, Joan Hodgman, Ronald Harper and Dennis McGinty.

REFERENCES

Astic, L. and Jouvet-Mounier, D. Mise en evidence
    du sommeil paradoxal in utero chez le cobaye.
    Comptes Rendus de la Academie de Science
    (Paris), 269: 2578-2581, 1969.

Baker, T. L. and McGinty, D. J. Reversal of cardio-
    pulmonary failure during active sleep in
    hypoxic kittens: Implications for Sudden
    Infant Death. Science, 198: 419-421, 1977.

Davis, H., Davis, P. A., Loomis, A. L., Harvey, N.
    and Hobart, G. Human brain potentials during
    the onset of sleep. Journal of Neurophysiology,
    1: 24-38, 1938.

Globus, G. G. Quantification of the sleep cycle
    as a rhythm. Psychophysiology, 7: 248-253,
    1970.

Harper, R. M., Hoppenbrouwers, T., Sterman, M. B.
    McGinty, D. J. and Hodgman, J. Polygraphic
    studies of normal infants during the first
    six months of life. I. Heart rate and varia-
    bility as a function of state. Pediatric
    Research, 10: 945-951, 1976.

Hoppenbrouwers, T., Harper, R. M., Hodgman, J. E.,
    Sterman, M. B. and McGinty, D. J. Polygraphic
    studies of normal infants during the first
    six months of life: II. Respiratory rate and
    variability as a function of state. Pediatric
    Research, in press, 1977.

Jouvet, M. Telencephalic and rhombencephalic
    sleep in the cat. In Nature of Sleep. Ciba
    Foundation Symposium, 1960, pp. 188-206.

Jouvet, M. Recherches sur les structures nervouses
    et mechanismes responsibles des differents
    phases du sommeil physiologique. Archives
    Italiannes de Biologie, 100: 125-206, 1962.

Jouvet, M. Etude de la dualite des etats de sommeil
    et des mecanismes de la phase paradoxale. In M.
    Jouvet (Ed.), Neurophysiologie des Etats de
    Sommeil. Centre National de la Recherche
    Scientifique, Paris, 1965, pp. 397-449.

Jouvet, M. Neurophysiology of the states of sleep. Physiological Reviews, 47(2): 117-177, 1967.

Kleitman, N. Sleep and Wakefulness. University of Chicago Press, Chicago, 1963, 552 pp.

Kleitman, N. and Engelmann, T. G. Sleep characteristics of infants. Journal of Applied Physiology, 6: 269-282, 1953.

Kripke, D. F. Ultradian rhythms in sleep and wakefulness. In Advances in Sleep Research, Vol. 1, Spectrum Publications, 1974, pp. 305-325.

Maloney, J. E. Respiratory periodicity in the foetal lamb. Presentation at: Research Reporting Workshop for NICHD Sudden Infant Death Syndrome Grantees and Contractors, Alexandria, VA., September, 1977.

Martin, C. B., Murata, Y., Petrie, R. H. and Parer, J. T. Respiratory movements in fetal rhesus monkeys. American Journal of Obstetrics and Gynaecology, 119: 939-948, 1974.

Orlandini, O., Sass-Kortsak, A. and Ebbs, J. Gamma globulin levels in normal infants. Pediatrics, 16: 575-584, 1955.

Othmer, E., Hayden, M. P. and Segelbaum, R. Encephalic cycles during sleep and wakefulness: A 24-hour pattern. Science, 164: 447-449, 1969.

Parmelee, A. H. and Stern, E. Development of states in infants. In C. D. Clemente, D. P. Purpura and F. E. Mayer (Eds.), Sleep and the Maturing Nervous System. Academic Press, New York, 1972 pp. 199-215.

Parmelee, A. H. Jr., Wenner, W. H. and Schulz, H. R. Infant sleep patterns from birth to 16 weeks of age. Journal of Pediatrics, 65: 576-582, 1964.

Patrick, J. Fetal respiration in babies who subsequently died of SIDS. In Proceedings of Research Reporting Workshop for NICHD Sudden Infant Death Syndrome Grantees and Contractors, Alexandria, VA, September, 1977.

Ruckebusch, Y.   Development of sleep and wake-
    fulness in the foetal lamb. Electroencephalo-
    graphy and Clinical Neurophysiology, 32: 119-
    128, 1972.

Schaffer, A. J., Markowitz, M. and Finberg, L.
    Diseases of the Newborn.   W. B. Saunders,
    Philadelphia, 1965, pp. 713-719.

Scheibel, M. E. and Scheibel, A. B.   Some structural
    and functional substrates of development in
    young cats.   In W. A. Himwich and H. E.
    Himwich (Eds.), The Developing Brain, Progress
    in Brain Research, Vol. 9., Elsevier, Amsterdam,
    1964, pp. 6-25.

Scheibel, M. E. and Scheibel, A. B.   Selected
    structural-functional correlations in post-
    natal brain.   In M. B. Sterman, D. J. McGinty
    and A. M. Adinolfi (Eds.) Brain Development
    and Behavior, Academic Press, New York, 1971,
    pp. 1-21.

Sterman, M. B.   Relationship of intrauterine fetal
    activity to maternal sleep stage.   Experimental
    Neurology, 4: 98-106, 1967.

Sterman, M. B.   The basic rest-activity cycle and
    sleep: Developmental considerations in man
    and cats.   In C. C. Clemente, D. P.   Purpura
    and F. E. Mayer (Eds.), Sleep and the Maturing
    Nervous System.   Academic Press, New York and
    London, 1972, pp. 175-197.

Sterman, M. B.   Sleep.   In L. DiCara (Ed.)
    Advances in Limbic and Autonomic Nervous
    System Research, Plenum Publishing Corporation,
    New York, 1974, pp. 395-417.

Sterman, M. B., Harper, R. M., Havens, B.,
    Hoppenbrouwers, T., McGinty, D. J. and Hodgman,
    J. E.   Quantitative analysis of infant EEG
    development during quiet sleep.   Electroence-
    phalography and Clinical Neurophysiology, 43:
    371-385, 1977.

Sterman, M. B., Hodgman, J. E., Hoppenbrouwers, T., Harper, R., Martin, C. B. and Siassi, B. Cardipulmonary patterns during quiet and active states in the fetus, newborn and infant. Sleep Research, 2: 79, 1973.

Sterman, M. B. and Hoppenbrouwers, T. The development of sleep-waking and rest-activity patterns from fetus to adult in man. In M. B. Sterman, D. J. McGinty and A. M. Adinolfi (Eds.), Brain Development and Behavior, Academic Press, New York, 1971, pp. 203-227.

Sterman, M. B., Lucas, E. A. and MacDonald, L. R. Periodicity within sleep and operant performance in the cat. Brain Research, 38: 327-341, 1972.

Usher, R. and McLean, F. Intrauterine growth of live-born caucasian infants at sea level: Standards obtained from measurements in seven dimensions of infants born between 25 and 44 weeks of gestation. Journal of Pediatrics, 74: 901-910, 1969.

A MOTIVATIONAL FUNCTION OF REM SLEEP

GERALD W. VOGEL

Emory University School of Medicine
Sleep Laboratory
Georgia Mental Health Institute
Atlanta, Georgia

INTRODUCTION

Many theories of REM sleep (RS) function have been proposed. A phylogenetic theory is that RS provides periodic activation and/or arousal to prepare a prey for "fight or flight" response to a predator (Snyder, 1965). An ontogenetic theory is that during infancy RS provides endogenous stimulation necessary for brain maturation (Roffwarg, et al., 1966). An oculomotor theory is that RS provides endogenous stimulation necessary for optimal performance of the brain mechanisms involved in binocular vision (Berger, 1969). Cognitive theories suggest that RS consolidates memory or facilitates new learning (Pearlman and Greenberg, 1968; Stern, 1969; Fishbein, 1969; 1970; Pearlman, 1971). As Feinberg and Evarts (1969) state "it should be noted that the functions proposed are not mutually exclusive". Nor is it likely that a complex brain state such as RS would have only one function, any more than waking has one function. The multiple processes associated with RS undoubtedly accomplish many functions or effects.

However, none of the above theories of RS explain the finding that REM sleep deprivation (RSD) improved endogenous depression (Vogel, et al., 1975). In this paper, I propose a motivational theory of RS to explain that finding. The motivational theory is not intended to preempt other RS theories. As implied above, it is simply a theory about one of several RS functions.

For expository purposes, I first present a synopsis of the theory. The supporting evidence follows the synopsis.

Synopsis

The idea that RS has a motivational function

Copyright © 1979 by Academic Press, Inc.
All rights of reproduction in any form reserved.
ISBN 0-12-222340-3

was instigated by the finding that RSD affects
motivated behavior in animals and in humans with
endogenous depression (Vogel, 1975; Vogel, et al.,
1975). In animals RSD increases such drive motivated behaviors as sex, aggression, pleasure seeking,
food seeking and grooming. Since decreases of these
behaviors are symptoms of endogenous depression, it
is not entirely surprising that RSD also improves
endogenous depression.

A motivational function of RS is inferred from
these observations that RSD increases drive motivated behavior. Since RS reverses this effect of
RSD, it follows - and this is the crux of the motivational theory - that RS decreases waking drive
motivated behavior.

The motivational theory includes a physiological section about how RSD increases drive motivated
behavior and how RS decreases that behavior. The
goal of that theoretical section is a parsimonious
physiological explanation of several aspects of
endogenous depression, viz, its clinical symptoms,
its RS abnormalities, its improvement by RSD, and
the RS correlates of its improvement by RSD.

Three observations form the basis of our physiological theory. First, RSD increases the waking
neural excitability of many brain structures (Vogel,
1975). Second, when RS is allowed after RSD, post-
RSD waking neural excitability decreases to pre-RSD
levels (Vogel, 1975). And third, during RS, profound
disinhibition augments neural firing rates in many
brain structures (Evarts, 1965; 1967).

These observations suggest that RSD increases
waking neural excitability by preventing neural
disinhibition and augmented neural firing rates
that occur during RS. Inversely, the observations
suggest that RS decreases waking neural excitability
in many brain structures because during RS, the
structures become disinhibited and have augmented
firing rates.

The theory also attempts to deal with the
duration of RSD effects. Increases of neural excitability caused by RSD are moderately persistent.
They last at least until the animal is allowed to
have RS and some effects may persist for a time
even after recovery RS (Vogel, 1975). Based on
findings discussed later, the theory proposes the
following explanation of the moderate persistence
of RSD effects. In addition to stimulating neural
excitability, RSD also correlatively stimulates a

linked, inhibitory mechanism (such as negative
feedback) that temporarily inhibits an abrupt discharge of the entire stimulated excitability. The
inhibitory mechanism postpones discharge of some
augmented excitability to a later time. Augmented
excitability is then gradually discharged as its
correlated augmented inhibition gradually diminishes. In short, RSD increases waking neural excitability by preventing neural discharge during sleep
and sustains the excitability by interfering with
its rapid discharge during waking.

Applied to animal drive motivated behavior,
the theory holds that prevention of periodic disinhibition and neural discharge during RSD increases
the waking excitability of a drive's neural substrate and thereby increases the waking drive. Inversely, the theory holds that disinhibition and
neural discharge during RS reduce the waking excitability of the drive's neural substrate and thereby reduce the waking drive.

Applied to endogenous depression, the physiological theory can coherently explain several aspects
of the disease in terms of the inverse relation
between waking drive motivated behavior and RS
neural disinhibition. (1) The RS abnormalities of
the disease are consistent with augmented neural
disinhibition during sleep. (2) Many clinical
symptoms of the disease (decreased sex, aggression,
pleasure seeking, food seeking, grooming) represent
large diminutions of the same animal drives that
are reduced by RS. Since large drive diminutions
can presumably result from augmented RS neural disinhibition, the clinical symptoms of depression, as
well as the RS abnormalities, may be caused by
augmented RS disinhibition. (3) Finally, RSD improves depression by reversing the physiological
effects of augmented disinhibition during RS. We
infer this because RSD improves depression to the
extent that it stimulates both neural excitability
and mechanisms that inhibit the abrupt discharge of
the stimulated excitability. Thus the theory's
upshot is that RSD improves depression to the extent
that the treatment counteracts the theoretical
cause of some salient features of depression. As
a result, the motivational theory of RS (including
its physiological section) may provide a consistent
explanation of many psychological and physiological
features of endogenous depression as well as of the

behavioral effects of RSD in animals and in humans
with endogenous depression.

EVIDENCE FOR THEORY

Motivational Effects of RS and RSD

The effect of RSD on several drive motivated
behaviors of animals has been studied and critically reviewed (Vogel, 1975). In rats, compared with
control procedures, RSD increased shock induced
fighting, the copulation rate of low baseline
copulators, and in animals given amphetamines,
sexual mountings and aggressive posturing (Morden,
et al., 1968a, Morden, et al., 1968b; Ferguson and
Dement, 1969). Also in rats, RSD lowered the threshold for, and increased the response rate of, intracranial self stimulation - presumably for an indicator of pleasure seeking behavior (Steiner and
Ellman, 1972). In less well controlled experiments
in cats, RSD increased sexual behavior, drive for
food and grooming behavior (Dement, 1965). When the
effect of RS after RSD was studied, the RS allowed
drive behavior to return toward pre-RSD levels
(Morden, et al., 1968a; Steiner and Ellman, 1972).
To summarize, in animals, RSD produced an increase
in the following drive motivated behaviors: aggressive and sexual activity, pleasure seeking, grooming
and food seeking. RS, on the other hand, reversed
the increase of drive motivated behavior caused by
RSD.

Neural Substrate of the Motivational Effects of RS and RSD

In animals, the effect of RSD on neural excitability has also been studied, and critically
reviewed (Vogel, 1975).
RSD decreased the electrical threshold for
seizures and prolonged the tonic phase of induced
convulsions (Cohen and Dement, 1965; 1968; Owen and
Bliss, 1970; Hartmann, et al., 1968; Cohen, et al.,
1970). In addition, RSD facilitated recovery of
cortical potentials evoked by external auditory
stimuli (Dewson, et al., 1967). RSD for seven days
increased entorhinal potentials evoked by single
shocks to the nearby cortex or to the pyriform, and
decreased sensory evoked potentials at the trige-
nimal nucleus and reticular formation (Satinoff,

et al., 1971). In the author's interpretation of
these last findings, RSD did "...not lead to a
general increase in neural excitability but rather
to paleocortical excitability and to an increase
in the inhibition responsible for sensory filtering". When the effect of RS after RSD was studied,
RS allowed indicators of neural excitability to
return to pre-RSD levels (Cohen and Dement, 1965;
Dewson, et al., 1967; Cohen et al., 1970; Satinoff,
et al., 1971). In general then, RSD increased
waking neural excitability in many, but not all,
brain structures that were studied; and RS reversed
these effects of RSD. To the best of my knowledge,
the effect of RSD on neural structures involved in
drive behavior has not been studied.

Nevertheless, when the behavioral and neural
studies are considered together, they suggest that
RSD stimulated drive motivated behavior by stimulating waking excitability of the neural structures
responsible for this behavior. Since RS reversed
these effects of RSD, we infer that RS reduced
waking drive motivated behavior by reducing the
waking neural excitability of the brain structures
responsible for this behavior.

Processes by which RS and RSD Affect Neural Excitability

We do not know how neural excitability is
reduced by RS or increased by RSD. Nevertheless,
it is plausible that to understand these processes,
our evidence should include findings about unit
(neuronal) activity during RS and RSD. To the best
of my knowledge, there are no studies of the effects
of RSD on unit activity. On the other hand, unit
activity during RS - as well as during NREM sleep
and wakefulness - was studied in a series of investigations pioneered by Evarts (1965; 1967). A
brief review of these studies follows.

Prior to Evarts' work, sleep was considered to
be a period of neural inactivity during which neurons
"rested". The hypothesized neural rest was thought
to be the physiological basis of the restorative
functions of sleep. Evarts' work refuted that
hypothesis. He and others found that neurons did
not become inactive during sleep (Evarts, 1965; 1967;
Rossi, et al., -961). The highest rates of unit
discharge frequency occurred during active wakefulness and RS. The lowest occurred during slow sleep

and quiet waking. Thus, in the switch from waking
to sleep, the salient change in unit activity was
not a reduction in average discharge frequency.
But unit activity did change in other ways. Evarts
found sleep-waking differences in the temporo-spatial
patterns of unit activity, in the ratio of evoked
to spontaneous unit activity, and in the discharge
rate differences between units. The temporal pattern
of spontaneous unit activity was regular during
waking, but during sleep it became irregular with,
high frequency bursts interrupted by relatively long
periods of unit silence. During RS the irregularity
was much greater than during slow sleep. The spatial
pattern of unit activity was a reciprocal discharge
of adjacent neurons during waking. During sleep,
adjacent neurons usually operated in unison. The
ratio of evoked to spontaneous discharge rate was
reduced during sleep compared with waking "a phenomenon which may be likened to a (decreased) in the
signal to noise ratio". Finally, in the switch
from waking to sleep, the discharge rate of different units became more alike. Units with a slow
waking discharge speeded up during sleep and units
with a fast waking discharge slowed down during
sleep.

     Evarts suggested that the neural changes in
the switch from waking to sleep occurred because
sleep was a period of generalized neural disinhibition (Evarts, 1965). He noted that Phillips had
previously shown that feedback disinhibition of
neurons was a possible explanation of the burst -
silence temporal pattern during sleep (Phillips,
1959). The exaggeration of this pattern during RS -
along with the large RS increase of discharge frequency - implied that neural dishinhibition was
maximum during RS. The sleep spatial pattern
(adjacent neurons discharge in unison rather than
reciprocally) and the small variance in neural discharge during sleep implied that during sleep the
neural disinhibition was widespread and generally
indiscriminate. Thus the observed waking-sleep
differences in unit activity were consistent with
increased unit disinhibition during sleep.

     Moreover, the sleep disinhibition hypothesis
was supported by the results of direct experimental
manipulations (Evarts, 1965; 1967). (1) In response
to stimulation of the lateral geniculate, the recovery cycle in the visual cortex was more depressed

in waking than sleep. (2) Stimulation of the lateral geniculate caused greater inhibition of spontaneous discharge in the visual cortex during waking
than during sleep. (3) In the visual cortex responses to the submaximal stimulation of the lateral
geniculate radiation increased from waking to sleep
but responses to supramaximal stimuli did not.
This suggested that during the submaximal stimulation, a greater subliminal fringe was recruited in
sleep than waking. (4) Long latency responses to
stimulation were more likely during waking than
during sleep, another finding consistent with greater disinhibition during sleep.

    To these experiments of Evarts, we may add two
additional supports for the view that sleep - and
in particular RS - is a period of profound neural
disinhibition. (1) A reduction of inhibition of
pyramidal tract cells was consistent with the tendency for epileptic attacks and myoclonus to be
precipitated by sleep. (2) Hobson and McCarley
(1975) showed that a large number of observations
and experimental manipulations were consistent with
a sleep onset disinhibition that became progressively greater during NREM sleep until maximum disinhibition was reached during RS.

    Taken together, these findings support the
conclusion that during RS, neural disinhibition
causes augmented neural discharge rates. To this
empirical conclusion, our theory adds the hypothesis
that the reduction of waking excitability produced
by RS is an effect of the neural disinhibition
during RS. The mechanism by which RS disinhibition
causes this waking effect is unknown. However, the
following sequence seems to be a plausible causal
chain: RS disinhibition causes an augmented RS
neural discharge rate which reduces waking neural
excitability.

    Applied to the neural effects of RSD, these
considerations suggest that RSD increases waking
neural excitability by preventing disinhibition and
thereby preventing intense neural discharge during
sleep. It therefore seems plausible that RSD increases waking neural excitability by preventing
an intense neural discharge during RS.

    A neural mechanism involved in sustaining the
effects of RSD is suggested by the relationship
between two aspects of REM rebound (the increase of
RS caused by RSD). We refer to the magnitude of
the rebound and to its temporal course. (Although

the former has been well studied, the latter has
not received attention). In healthy subjects, the
rebound is postponed beyond the first REM period so
that most of it occurs in later REM periods or even
after the first recovery night (Dement, 1964;
Vogel, 1977). The postponement of REM rebound
suggests that increased RS inhibition operates
during the first REM period to prevent the occurrence of some of the RSD stimulated RS. Without such
inhibition, presumably all the excess RS generated
by RSD would occur during the first REM period. In
other words, a postponed REM rebound suggests that
RSD stimulates both RS generation (hence the REM
rebound) and a temporary RS inhibition (hence the
REM postponement) that prevents uninterrupted complete discharge of the excess RS stimulated by RSD.
Since our laboratory found that total rebound correlated positively with rebound after the first REM
period, we conclude that RSD correlatively stimulates RS and a linked, inhibitory mechanism (such
as a negative feedback loop) (Vogel, et al., 1977).
As the strength of the linked inhibitory mechanism
wanes over time, more of the rebound is discharged.
Applying these mechanisms to other neural structures,
we suggest that RSD increases waking neural excitability by preventing neural discharge during sleep
and sustains the waking excitability by interferr-
ing with its rapid and complete discharge during
waking.

Let us now use this neural theory to understand
how RS and RSD affect animal drive motivated behavior. In summary, the theory holds that prevention of periodic disinhibition and neural discharge
during RSD increases the waking excitability of a
drive's neural substrate and thereby increases the
waking drive. Inversely, the theory holds that
disinhibition and neural discharge during RS reduce
the waking excitability of the drive's neural substrate and thereby reduce the waking drive. In the
next section, this theory is applied to an understanding of several aspects of endogenous depression.

Application of the Motivational RS Theory to Endo-
genous Depression

Typical symptoms of endogenous depression include decreases of libido, aggressiveness, appetite
grooming behavior and pleasure seeking (Mendels and

Cochrane, 1968). Indeed, it is possible that the
mood disturbance of depression, the dejection, is an
amalgam of a loss of interest in all these elemental
bodily activities. Be that as it may, it is clear
that the above symptoms of endogenous depression
represent large diminutions of the same drives that
in animals are reduced by RS. More precisely, and
in accordance with the proposed neural theory, the
depressive symptoms represent large diminutions of
the same animal drives that are reduced by augmented
neural disinhibition during RS. This suggests the
hypothesis that symptoms of endogenous depression
are a result of excessive neural disinhibition during
RS. This suggests the hypothesis that symptoms of
endogenous depression are a result of excessive
neural disinhibition during RS.

Recent findings in our laboratory support that
hypothesis (Vogel, et al., 1977). In comparing
depressives and age-insomnia matched, nondepressed
controls, we found RS abnormalities in depression
that were consistent with excessive neural disinhibition during RS. The depressive-control comparisons
were made both before and after RSD. We first describe the RS abnormalities in endogenous depression
and then show how they were consistent with excessive
neural disinhibition.

Compared with the controls, the depressives
had low REM latency, high REM frequency and abnormalities in the temporal distribution of RS. The last
abnormalities are easier to describe after RSD than
before, when they were less obvious. On the first
recovery night after RSD, the depressives had longer
first REM periods and less subsequent RS than the
controls. Since total REM sleep and total sleep
time were not significantly different in the two
groups, the depressives simply had more REM sleep
early and less REM sleep later. Before RSD, the
same phenomena occurred but not on every baseline
night. But when the longest first REM period of
each subject in the two groups was compared, depressive first REM periods were significantly longer.
This was not so for lesser ranked first REM periods.
Moreover, on the nights of each subject's longest
first REM periods, subsequent mean REM periods
(though not subsequent total REM sleep) were significantly shorter in depressives than controls.
Finally, during the baseline, first REM period
duration and subsequent REM sleep duration varied
significantly more in depressives than controls.

In short, the salient depressive RS abnormalities
were low REM latency, high REM frequency and a
variable tendency for more REM sleep early in the
night and less later in the night, a tendency which
was exacerbated by RSD.

To determine whether these RS abnormalities
were consistent with increased neural disinhibition
during RS, we used a physiologic model of the
mammalian sleep oscillator which explicitly took
neural disinhibition into account. Authored by
Hobson and McCarley (1975), this model proposed
that the cyclic alternation of NREM and REM sleep
resulted from the reciprocal interaction of two
pontine neuronal groups; one that generated RS and
one that inhibited RS. In this oscillator, reduced
activity of the inhibitor, i.e., disinhibition, was
necessary for RS.

Without discussing the details of the oscillator
- or of the controversy about the anatomical location of its parts - we consider how a Hobson-McCarley
oscillator can explain the depressive RS abnormalities. McCarley and Hobson (1975) made this
possible by showing that the physiological oscillator
could be mathematically modeled by a pair of simultaneous differential equations, the Lotka-Volterra
equations. When a RS generator strength and a RS
inhibitor strength were inserted as constants in
these equations, their solutions provided durations
of REM and NREM parts of the cycle. Using the
computer to obtain numerical solutions to these
nonlinear equations, we found an inhibitor strength
and a generator strength which produced a cycle with
NREM - REM proportions similar to the first cycle
of the nondepressed controls (Vogel, et al., 1977).
We then found that reduction of the generator and
inhibitor strengths (reduced inhibition represented
greater disinhibition), produced a cycle like the
depressive first cycle with low REM latency and a
long first REM period. Indeed, the first cycles of
the actual depressives and controls were remarkably
similar to their respective mathematical models.
Specifically, the ratio of depressive to control
REM latency and the ratio of depressive to control
first REM period duration were almost identical in
the actual subjects and in their mathematical models.
Thus, augmented neural disinhibition is consistent
with the low REM latency and long first REM periods
seen in the depressives. To determine whether
augmented disinhibition would produce more variable

first REM periods (as seen in the depressives), we
introduced several small perturbations of inhibitory strengths in the depressive and control mathematical models. Over a range of several inhibitory
perturbations, the same perturbation in the depressives and in the controls produced a greater
change in the depressive first REM period than in
the control. Hence, increased neural disinhibition
can also explain the greater variability of the
depressive first REM period. Thus, in terms of the
Hobson-McCarley oscillator, the depressive first
cycle abnormalities are consistent with increased
neural disinhibition during RS.

Although other depressive RS abnormalities
(increased REM frequency and decreased later REM%)
are not modeled by the Lotka-Volterra equations,
Aserinsky's work suggests that these abnormalities,
as well as those in the first cycle, are a reflection of augmented neural disinhibition (Aserinsky,
1969). In a study of the extended sleep of healthy
young adults, Aserinsky found that during the first
four or five successive cycles, REM periods usually
became progressively longer and REM frequencies
usually became progressively higher. REM periods
after the fourth or fifth became shorter while REM
frequencies remained high.

Our previous application of the Hobson-McCarley
oscillator showed that greater RS disinhibition
produced longer REM periods. Applied to Aserinsky's
findings, this means that successive REM periods became progressively longer (and more intense) because
RS disinhibition became progressively greater. At
about the fourth REM period, disinhibition reached
the maximum, making REM period duration maximum
and NREM period minimum. After that, we postulate
that an unknown effect of the very long REM period
(e.g. temporary transmitter deficiency) made subsequent REM periods shorter but their REM frequency
remained intense because of the persistently high
RS disinhibition.

The sequence of cycles in Aserinsky's subjects
may shed light on the depressive sequence of cycles.
The depressive sequence, beginning with their first
REM period, resembled the sequence in Aserinsky's
subjects beginning with their fourth or fifth REM
period. In each case, after a very short NREM
period (REM latency for the depressives), a long REM
period with high REM frequency was followed by
shorter REM periods with continued high REM

frequency. Thus, the depressives on nights of
maximum first REM periods, began sleep with their
sequence of cycles like the control sequence after
six to eight hours of sleep. Since the latter was
consistent with augmented RS disinhibition, the
similar depressive sequences of REM periods was
also consistent with augmented RS disinhibition.
Thus, the Hobson-McCarley oscillator and Aserinsky's
extended sleep phenomenon suggest that the RS abnormalities of endogenous depression were caused by
augmented neural disinhibition during RS. This conclusion is consistent with the previous one that
augmented RS neural disinhibition also caused many
clinical symptoms of endogenous depression.

Finally, we suggest an explanation of how RSD
improved endogenous depression. Two correlations
are relevant here. In the depressives treated by
RSD, clinical improvement correlated positively
with postponed REM rebound and with REM pressure
(RS after RSD divided by RS before RSD). As discussed previously, postponed REM rebound indicated
the RS inhibition that operated during the first
REM period to postpone the rebound. Thus improvement correlated with the RS inhibition (or reversal
of disinhibition) stimulated by RSD. On the other
hand, REM pressure, the augmentation of RS stimulated by RSD, indicated an augmented neural excitability in the RS system. It seems plausible that
the RSD augmentation of neural excitability in the
RS system was a rough indicator of how strongly RSD
augmented neural excitability in other neural
systems. Thus, the correlations of improvement were
consistent with the view that RSD improved depression
by stimulating a RS inhibition (or reducing a RS
disinhibition) that prevented the sudden, complete
discharge of the stimulated excitability.

It is noteworthy that REM pressure and postponed RS correlated positively with each other. The
correlation implies that in the RS neural system,
the mechanisms responsible for excitability and for
inhibition of the system were linked. One possible
kind of linkage was a negative feedback loop, such
as proposed by Hobson and McCarley in their reciprocal interaction oscillator (Hobson, et al., 1975).
In any event, in this linked system, RSD stimulated
inhibition (postponed rebound) less in the depressives than in the controls but its stimulation of
excitability (REM pressure) was not significantly

different in the two groups. Like the baseline
depressive control differences, this again suggests
that the "damage" in the depressive oscillator was
primarily in a RS inhibitor.

In conclusion, the motivational theory of RS
offers a consistent explanation of several aspects
of endogenous depression. It can explain many
clinical symptoms and REM sleep abnormalities as a
result of RS augmented neural disinhibition and its
consequence, viz, reduced waking neural excitability. It then consistently explains that RSD improved
depression by reversing and counteracting these
effects of augmented neural disinhibition.

OTHER IMPLICATIONS OF THE MOTIVATIONAL THEORY OF RS

The motivational theory raises the question of
why RSD has not clearly affected drive motivation
in healthy, nondepressed humans (Vogel, 1975). Two
possible (and not incompatible) answers are suggested by relevant findings. One is that in humans -
and possibly in all primates - there is an upper
limit or ceiling on the excitability that can be
stimulated by RSD. Consistent with this is the
finding that antidepressant drugs, which suppress
RS, do not usually have a remarkable effect on drive
behaviors in nondepressed humans. Another possible
answer might lie in the duration of RSD required to
produce an effect on human, as contrasted with
animal, drive motivation. In endogenous depression,
about three weeks of RSD were required to increase
drive motivated behavior. Nondepressed humans have
not been REM sleep deprived for that long. Thus
the motivational effects of RS may require several
weeks before they become noticeable in humans.
Indeed, the long time scale might have adaptive
value in that it implies a relative stability in
the mechanisms that sustain these vital behaviors.

That RS has an adaptive value seems obvious
from its presence in all placental mammals. The
motivational theory suggests that the drive reduction by RS should have an adaptive value in these
phylogenetically higher organisms. One possible
value might be that RS tames or modulates drive
oriented behavior so as to permit higher organisms
behavioral flexibility in the presence of drive
motivations. The flexibility would permit an adaptively specific responsiveness in the pursuit of
drive gratification. It would include a capacity

to delay drive gratification in order to respond
with adaptive variability to environmental exi-
gencies presented during the drive motivation. Put
in slightly different terms, the presence of RS
allows higher organisms to be less driven, less
relentless, less stereotyped and more adaptively
specific in response to primitive drives or instinctual motivation. Thus it may be that modern sleep
research on laboratory animals and human depressives
has supported the old, occasionally derogated, psychological view that dreams discharge instinctual tensions (Freud, 1953).

REFERENCES

Aserinsky, E. The maximal capacity for sleep: Rapid
     eye movement density as an index of sleep
     satiety. Biological Psychiatry, 1: 147-159,
     1959.

Berger, R. J. Oculomotor control: A possible func-
     tion of REM sleep. Psychological Review, 76:
     144-164, 1969.

Carroll, BJ.Curtis, C. G., and Mendels, J. Neuro-
     endocrine regulation in depression. I. Limbic
     system - adrenocortical dysfunction. Archives
     of General Psychiatry, 33: 1039-1044, 1976.

Carroll, B. J., Curtis, C. G. and Mendels, J.
     Neuroendocrine regulation in depression. I.
     Discrimination of depressed from nondepressed
     patients. Archives of General Psychiatry, 33:
     1051-1058, 1976.

Cohen, H. B., Dement, W. C. Sleep: Changes in
     threshold to electroconvulsive shock in rats
     after deprivation of "paradoxical" phase.
     Science, 150: 1318-1319, 1965.

Cohen, H. B., Dement, W. C. Electrically induced
     convulsions in REM deprived mice: Prolongation
     of the tonic phase, absgracted. Psychophysio-
     logy, 4: 381, 1968.

Cohen, H. B., Thomas, J., and Dement, W. C. Sleep styles, REM deprivation, and electroconvulsive threshold in the cat. Brain Research, 19: 317-321, 1970.

Dement, W. C. Experimental dream studiesn. In: Masserman, J. (ed.) Science and Psychoanalysis, New York, Grune and Stratton, Vol. 7, 1964, pp. 128-162.

Dement, W. C. Recent studies on the biological role of REM sleep. American Journal of Psychiatry, 122: 404-408, 1965.

Dewson, J. H. III, Dement, W. C., Wagener, T. E., and Nobel, K. Rapid eye movement sleep deprivation: A central neural change during wakefulness. Science, 156: 403-406, 1967.

Evarts, E. V. Neuronal activity in vusual and motor cortex during sleep and waking. In: Jouvet, M. (Ed.) Neurophysiologie de Etats de Sommeil, Paris, Centre-National de la Recherche Scientifique, 1965, pp. 189-209.

Evarts, E. V. Activity of individual cerebral neurons during sleep and arousal. In: Kety, S. S., Evarts, E. V., William, H. L. (eds.), Sleep and altered states of consciousness, Baltimore, Williams and Wilkins, 1967, pp. 316-336.

Feinberg, I. Evarts, E. V. Changing concepts of the function of sleep: discovery of intense brain activity during sleep calls for revision of hypotheses as to its function. Biological Psychiatry, 1: 331-348, 1969.

Ferguson, J., Dement, W. C. The behavioral effects of amphetamines on REM deprived rats. Journal of Psychiatric Research, 7: 111-118, 1969.

Fishbein, W. The effects of paradoxical sleep deprivation during the retention interval on long term memory. Abstract of the Association for the Psychophysiological Study of Sleep, Boston, 1969.

Fishbein, W. Interference with conversion of memory from short term to long term storage by partial sleep deprivation. Communications in Behavioral Biology, 5: 171-176, 1970.

Freud, S. The Interpretation of Dreams. London, The Hogarth Press, 1953, Vol. 4 and 5, The Standard Edition of the Complete Psychological Works of Sigmund Freud.

Hartman, E., Marcus, J., and Lernoff, A. The sleep-dream cycle and convulsive threshold. Psychonomic Science, 13: 141-142, 1968.

Hobson, J. A., McCarley, R. S. and Wyzinski, P. W. Sleep cycle oscillation: Reciprocal discharge by two brainstem neuronal groups. Science, 189: 55-58, 1975.

Mendels, J. and Cochrane, C. The nosology of depression: the endogenous-reactive concept. American Journal of Psychiatry, 124: 1-11 (suppl), 1968.

McCarley, R. W. and Hobson, J. A. Neuronal excitability modulation over the sleep cycle: a structural and mathematical model. Science, 189: 58-60, 1975.

Morden, B., Conner, R., Mitchell, G., Dement, W., and Levine, S. Effects of rapid eye movement (REM) sleep deprivation on shock induced fighting. Physiology and Behavior, 3: 425-432, 1968 a.

Morden, B., Mullins, R., Levine, S., Cohen, H., Dement, W. Effect of REMS deprivation on the mating behavior of male rats, abstracted. Psychophysiology, 5: 241-242, 1968 b.

Owen, M., and Bliss, E. Sleep loss and cortical excitability. American Journal of Physiology, 218: 171-173, 1970.

Pearlman, C. and Greenberg, R. Effect of REM deprivation on retention of avoidance learning in rats. Abstract of the Association for the Psychophysiological Study of Sleep, Denver, 1968.

Pearlman, C. Latent learning impaired by REM sleep deprivation. Psychonomic Science, 25: 135-136, 1971.

Phillips, C. Actions of antidromic pyramidal volleys on single Betz calls in the cat. Quarterly Journal of Experimental Physiology, 44: 1-25, 1959.

Roffwarg, H. P., Muzio, J. N., and Dement, W. C. Ontogenetic development of the human sleep-dream cycle. Science, 152: 604-619, 1966.

Rossi, G. F., Favale, E., Hara, T., Guisanni, A., and Sacco, G. Researches of the nervous mechanisms underlying deep sleep in the cat. Archives of Italian Biology, 99: 280-292, 1961.

Sachar, E., Hellman, L., Roffwarg, H., Halpern, F., Fukushima, D. and Gallagher, T. Disrupted 24-hour patterns of cortisol secretion in psychotic depression. Archives of General Psychiatry, 28: 19-24, 1973.

Satinoff, E., Drucker-Colin, R. R. and Hernandez-Peon, R. Paleocortical excitability and sensory filtering during REM sleep deprivation. Physiology and Behavior, 7: 103-106, 1971.

Snyder, F. Progress in the new biology of dreaming. American Journal of Psychiatry, 122: 377-390, 1965.

Steiner, S. S. and Ellman, S. J. Relation between REM sleep and intracranial self stimulation. Science, 177: 1122-1124, 1972.

Stern, W. C. Effects of REM sleep deprivation upon the acquisition and maintainence of learned behavior in the rat. Abstract of the Association for the Psychophysiological Study of Sleep, Boston, 1969.

Vogel, G. W. A review of REM sleep deprivation. Archives of General Psychiatry, 32: 749-761, 1975.

Vogel, G. W., Augustine, F., McAbee, R., and Thurmond,
    A. New findings about how REM sleep depriva-
    tion improves depression. Unpublished manu-
    script and read before the Association for the
    Psychophysiological Study of Sleep, Houston,
    1977.

WHAT CAN INSOMNIACS TEACH US ABOUT
THE FUNCTIONS OF SLEEP ?

PETER HAURI

Department of Psychiatry
Dartmouth Medical School
Hanover, New Hampshire

Inviting a behavioral sleep clinician to this symposium was probably motivated by the hope that a study of insomnia might shed some new light on the function of sleep. This assumption is based on a time-honored method in physiology: When trying to discern the function of an organ, system, or pathway, take it away and see what happens to the rest of the organism. To state it clearly at the outset, studying the lack of sleep has not given us a clear answer regarding the function of sleep. However, I think such a study can clarify some issues involved in this symposium, and it might clear up some misconceptions.

Before starting, some introductory comments:
(1) It seems logical that sleep has **many** functions, not **a** function. What, one might ask conversely, is the function of wakefulness? Although one might find some over-arching philosophical principle as the function of wakefulness, such as "survival", or "preservation of the genes", such a statement would be trite and of little help toward a scientific understanding of wakefulness. A list of many functions of wakefulness would help more, together with an enumeration of the various mechanisms by which each function is accomplished.

(2) It is obvious that there are at least two types of sleep. All but the most primitive of mammals have developed alternations between REM and NREM sleep. This suggests that each of the two basic sleep states might have different functions. However, in this paper, the typical mixture of sleep stages usually obtained by humans will be considered, without separating REM functions from those of NREM.

(3) Functions of sleep can probably be found on many different levels, from molecules up to the

Copyright © 1979 by Academic Press, Inc.
All rights of reproduction in any form reserved.
ISBN 0-12-222340-3

total behavior of the organism. This paper is
concerned with relatively global aspects of mood,
performance, and ANS activity.

4. Sleep and wakefulness are mutually interacting and cyclic phenomena, each affecting the
other. It seems impossible to disentangle effects
of sleep on wakefulness from effects of wakefulness
on sleep. Each can be both cause and effect of the
other. Maybe we should not try to understand the
function of sleep, but rather the function of the
rhythmic alternations between sleep and wakefulness.

Definitions

Optimal Sleep Requirement: There is evidence
that there exists an optimal amount of sleep for
each person at any given time. Sleeping less, or
more, than this optimum has deleterious effects on
waking mood and performance (Globus, 1969; Taub et
al., 1971).

Hypsosomnia: A hyposomniac is a person who functions optimally with very few hours of sleep
(Stuss et al., 1975).

Total Sleep Deprivation: All sleep of one or
more nights is artificially removed from a person
who could sleep normally if he were not part of the
experiment.

Selective Sleep Stage Deprivation: Certain
sleep stages, but not others, are artificially
removed.

Sleep Curtailment: A person is forced to
sleep less than would be optimal for him. Within
the short time allotted, he can sleep in whatever
stage comes naturally.

Insomnia: A person is unable to obtain his
optimal amount of sleep, even though he gives himself enough time in bed. The absolute number of
hours slept is inconsequential for this definition
of insomnia. A person might sleep 3 hours and not
be an insomniac because he does not need more
sleep. Another might sleep 8 hours and still be
an insomniac because, over an extended period of
time, he would function better if he were to sleep
10 hours.

The distinctions between the different forms
of lack of sleep are clearer, and the general
results found for sleep are foreshadowed somewhat
in an analogy with food and hunger. A hyposomniac
is analogous to somebody who functions optimally

when eating very few calories. There is no problem.
Total sleep deprivation is akin to absolute fasting.
Selective sleep stage deprivation is akin to eating
a specific, probably deficient, and somewhat
restricted diet. Sleep curtailment is similar to
chronic under-nutrition or semi-starvation. Finally, insomnia seems akin to anorexia nervosa, or to
some chronic malabsorption syndromes. The food is
available, but somehow it does not enter the blood-
stream.
        Let us now see what the various types of lack
of sleep can tell us about the functions of sleep.

Hyposomnia

        Whether hyposomniacs have a personality type
separate and distinct from long sleepers is still
a matter of debate. Hartmann et al. (1972) and Wagner
and Mooney (1975) believe that they do, while Webb
and Friel (1971) do not. However, all accept the
following facts:
        1. Very short sleep is quite compatible with
psychologically adequate functioning in some people.
        2. Nobody has found people or any other
mammals who can function entirely without sleep
(except for a case of Morvan's chorea reported by
Fischer-Perroudon et al., 1974). It appears that
a certain minimal level of sleep is biologically
necessary in mammals.
        3. Beyond a certain minimum amount, sleep
requirements vary widely, both between species and
among members of the same species. This variation
is not, however, open to free choice. Rather,
different humans apparently require different
amounts of sleep.

Total Sleep Deprivation

        The main, immediate effect of total sleep de-
privation is an increased drive to sleep. This
is analogous to the situation with food: skipping
a few meals usually increases our hunger quite dramatically, without initially causing noteworthy
physiological changes or medical problems.
        There is one important difference between
food and sleep (Rechtschaffen, personal communication). Food can be withheld from the outside.

Sleep is generated from within. Thus, when sleep
deprived, the body soon starts "snitching" a few
seconds of "mini-sleep". This means that short
lapses of attention occur, during which the EEG
shows drowsy or sleep waves. These episodes of
"mini-sleep" increase in duration and number with
sleep deprivation until, within about 10 days, it
becomes very hard to say from the EEG, or from
the person's behavior, whether he is actually
asleep or awake.

Mood during total sleep deprivation follows
a circadian rhythm and is generally worst during
times when one normally would be sleeping. Besides
an increase in fatigue, there is increased irritability and aggressiveness in both animals and man.
Humans report that almost anything takes greater
effort to accomplish after sleep deprivation; they
are generally serious, listless, and grim. Spontaneity is missing, and people feel washed out,
depleted, without reserves.

Aggressiveness and irritability can probably
be explained as the results of thwarting the sleep
drive, because both behaviors are also seen when
thwarting the hunger drive during starvation, or
when undergoing general stress. Other mood
aspects, however, such as the grim listlessness, the
feeling of depletion, etc., seem to be unique to
sleep deprivation. While most mood scales measure
primarily an increase in depression, calling the
mood after sleep deprivation "depression" is probably an error, due mainly to the technical limitations of currently available mood scales that were
developed to assess psychiatrically relevant waking
moods. In any case, anybody who has been seriously,
psychiatrically depressed on some occasions, and
purely sleep deprived on others, will attest to the
fact that the two mood states are different.

The initial decrements in performance after
total sleep deprivation can probably be ascribed to
the lapses of attention when taking mini-sleeps.
Later on, there do seem to be genuine decreases in
perceptual, cognitive, and psychomotor capabilities
(Pasnau et al., 1968).

Personality disorganization following sleep
deprivation is smaller than originally expected.
Nevertheless, there are bona fide transient ego
disrupt;ions (Pasnau et al., 1968), and periods of

disorientation, paranoid feelings, and occasional
episodes of losing emotional control.

Functioning of the ANS shows either a mixed
picture of activation/deactivation (Naitoh et al.,
1971, a), or arousal in the ANS (Johnson et al.,
1965). In any case, ANS functioning is clearly
disturbed. In addition, small changes in neurological functioning, such as a fine hand tremor,
a difficulty in focusing the eyes, and increased
sensitivity to pain, etc., are consequences of
sleep deprivation (Ross, 1965; Kollar et al., 1968).
Naitoh et al. (1971, b), also found a significant
reduction in "contingent negative variation" in the
EEG after sleep deprivation, suggesting lack of
"attentiveness" or expectancy (Walter et al., 1964).
Although these deficits are not life-threatening,
they do indicate that something went awry in the
nervous system which cannot be explained by a purely
behavioral-adaptational model or a psychological
drive to sleep.

Surprisingly, in many physiological and psychological variables, the maximum disruptive effects
of sleep deprivation are found within 2 to 5 days.
Some variables level off after that, others return
to baseline, while still others deteriorate further.
One might speculate that the mini-sleeps, which
gradually increase during prolonged sleep deprivation, are giving the body enough "bits of sleep"
to maintain a certain low level of functioning.

The changes caused by experimental sleep deprivation are discussed here in some detail to counteract the often heard statement that sleep deprivation does nothing much except increase the desire
to sleep. This is not true. To recapitulate, it:

1. causes profound mood disturbances;
2. causes heavy performance decrements;
3. results in temporary, but nevertheless
   real personality changes;
4. disturbs ANS and other neurological functions.

Deprivation of Specific Sleep Stages

Although experts still debate the issue, a
fair amount of evidence is accumulating that REM
sleep deprivation has different effects from delta
sleep deprivation. While performance on objective

work tasks seems disturbed to about the same degree
by both types of deprivation (Johnson, 1973), mood
states show differential effects.

Both in animals and in man, REM sleep deprivation seems to energize basic drives, or to weaken
control over these drives (Zarcone et al., 1974).
Fantasy life and some other higher mental functions
seem specifically affected (Cartwright, 1977).
Vogel et al. (1975) give convincing evidence suggesting that REM deprivation is as powerful an antidepressant as many drugs commonly used against depression.

Fewer studies have been carried out on delta
sleep deprivation. Agnew et al. (1967) suggest
that delta sleep deprivation made the subjects less
physically comfortable than REM deprivation. These
patients complained about vague physical symptoms
and about changes in bodily feeling. Moldofsky
and Scarisbrick (1976) found that delta sleep deprivation resulted in more musculoskeletal symptoms
and increased sensitivity to pain in joints and
muscles than did REM deprivation, and they suggest,
as does Hartmann (1973), that delta sleep is involved in the restoration of physical functioning.

Deprivation of either REM sleep or delta sleep
cannot be carried out in a vacuum. Influencing
one sleep stage influences the others, and there
is the possibility that basic phenomena from one
stage will "spill over" into others (Dement, 1972).
Nevertheless, the above evidence does suggest that
delta sleep is related to somatic recovery, while
REM sleep has something to do with the recovery of
higher mental functions. Blood flow measures
support such a view. During delta sleep blood
flow is directed mainly to the muscles, while cerebral arteries are constricted. During REM sleep
cerebral blood flow increases, while blood flow to
the large skeletal muscles is constricted (Townsend
et al., 1973; Hauri, 1966). It seems unlikely that
this switching in blood allocation is entirely without reason.

Concerning the functions of sleep, a purely
behavioral-adaptational model cannot account for
these differential effects of specific sleep stage
deprivation. If the main goal of sleep were to
keep the organism from responding, one uniform
state of hypoarousal would be quite satisfactory.

Sleep Curtailment

Few people undergo many consecutive nights of
total sleep deprivation, or specific deprivations
of individual stages. Most, however are quite
familiar with the effects of partial sleep deprivation, i.e., with the curtailment of sleep to very
few hours for a few weeks or months. Thus, it
seems unnecessary to document the subjectively
quite profound changes in mood after some nights
of curtailed sleep. This change of mood does not
seem to be a reaction to the acute disturbance of
the sleep/wake rhythm. Johnson and MacLeod (1973)
found that, even after weeks and months of sleep
curtailment to 5 and 4 hours per night, their
subjects still felt less happy, less friendly, less
energetic, and more fatigued than when they could
sleep ad lib.

According to Wilkinson et al. (1966), objectively assessed performance is quite sensitive to
sleep curtailment. In general, Wilkinson et al.
feel that effects of 3-½ hours deprivation per
night are clearcut and appear on the first or second
day following curtailment. If more prolonged
periods of curtailment are used, effects of 1-½
hours sleep loss per night can also be demonstrated.
Similarly, Webb (1975) found evidence of a performance decrement after the seventh and eighth nights
in students being restricted to 3 hours of sleep per
night, and a decrease in performance on a vigilance
task in students placed on a 5-½hour sleep schedule
for 8 weeks. However, Webb (1975) seems to dismiss
his own findings by claiming that "it was more a
matter of motivation than capacity". Why should
motivational defects be less real or important than
defects in capacity?

Taub and Berger (1976) suggest that the
absolute amounts of sleep may not be as crucial to
subsequent mood and performance as the disruption
of the 24-hours sleep-wakefulness cycle. Five
different conditions were assessed: habitual sleep
(9.5 to 10.5 hours), habitual sleep advanced 3
hours, habitual sleep delayed 3 hours, extended
sleep (3 hours added), and curtailed sleep (3 hours
substracted). Each experimental condition produced
an approximately equivalent decline in vigilance,
performance, and subjective arousal. However, the
results of Taub and Berger are based on only one
night in each condition. Quite likely, reactions

to one disturbed night might be the same no matter
what the type of disturbance, while reactions would
start to vary if people were kept in each condition
for more than just one night. In addition, even
in their own data, reactions to the different conditions were not totally equal. Furthermore, it
is scientifically impossible to prove equivalence
of results. Mood scales that are more sensitive
to sleep deprivation states might have found differences where the scales that were used did not.
Finally, Taub and Berger's conclusion disagrees
with the findings of Johnson and MacLeod (1973),
discussed earlier, which showed the typical deprivation moods after months of curtailed sleep stably
set within the circadian rhythm.

In sum, studies on curtailed sleep support the
studies reviewed earlier that lack of enough sleep
results in a specific dysphoric mood and in performance decrements.

Insomnia

Entering the realm of clinical insomnia, we
now leave the relatively solid experimental grounds
of laboratory deprived sleep with its rigid schedules, exact regimes, and sensitive performance
tests. As discussed earlier, insomnia cannot be
defined as a certain small number of hours slept
per night. Rather, it seems that each person has
an individually optimal sleep requirement.
Insomnia is then defined as a chronic inability to
obtain that optimal number of hours, even though
the individual spends enough time in bed.

To document objectively that somebody is an
insomniac is very difficult. One would first have
to record the person's usual amount of sleep, and
his daytime performance and mood. One would then
have to increase his sleep somehow (hopefully without medication) and document that with increased
sleep comes improved daytime mood and functioning.
This would all have to be averaged over a number of
nights, because functioning during a certain day
is not rigidly related to sleep on the one previous
night.

Because the exact laboratory demonstration
that somebody is an insomniac is technically so
cumbersome, one usually depends on the patients'
subjective statement that they feel they could

function better if they could sleep better. However, this is a very tenuous basis on which to diagnose insomnia. Personality traits such as hypochondriasis, denial, and repression play important roles in making the crucial statements, without being directly related to insomnia.

The reasons for insomnia are numerous and complex. In a recent survey of 141 patients studied at the Dartmouth Sleep Clinic, we found that about 1/3 of the insomniacs clearly showed serious psychiatric disturbances. Medical problems, such as sleep apneas, myoclonus, pain, etc. were the reason for insomnia in about 1/6 of our patients. In the remaining 50%, mild psychological disturbances such as anxiety, tension, or mild depression were usually present, but they seemed too weak to explain by themselves the relatively serious insomniacs. Rather, maladaptive, learned behavior patterns (bad habits) seemed to play important roles in many of these latter insomniacs (Hauri, 1976).

Proportions from other labs vary, but nobody argues the point that there are many and often totally different etiologies for the final common problem of insomnia. These etiologies need not concern us in detail here; they have been reviewed adequately in a number of publications (Kales and Kales, 1974; Hauri, 1975; Williams and Karacan, 1975; etc.).

In view of the extreme etiological heterogeneity of insomnia, it seems surprising that anything at all can be said about "the insomniacs" as a group. Nevertheless, a fair number of studies have been able to adequately characterize the majority of insomniacs, both on psychological and physiological levels. The fact that most insomniacs are psychologically and physiologically quite alike when their basic etiologies are so different suggests that the similarities among them are related to lack of sleep, the only common feature in this very heterogeneous group.

Almost without exception, and in marked contrast to hyposomniacs, insomniacs are characterized by dysphoric mood. Indeed, Kales et al. (1976) found that the MMPI Scale 2 was one of the highest three scales in about 70% of their insomniacs. This scale relates to worry, discouragement, low self esteem, and lack of comfort. People scoring high on it tend to be seen as silent, withdrawn,

evasive, timid, and inhibited. Coursey et al.
(1975), and Monroe (1967), among others, found
similar elevations of Scale 2.

      Based on clinical work, I personally feel
that the dysphoric mood described by insomniacs
is not akin to depression, although the words used
are the same, (listlessness, lack of spontaneity,
feeling drained and "washed out", depleted, and
without reserves). Most insomniacs describe a
feeling of being heavily slowed down, as if working
in an environment filled with molasses rather than
air. These feelings are quite similar to the feelings volunteers describe after total sleep deprivation for a few days, as discussed earlier.

      There is little question that general psycho-
pathology, as measured by the MMPI, the EPI, and
similar scales, is high in insomniacs. This was
first demonstrated by Monroe (1967) and later
replicated by Karacan et al. (1973), Coursey et al.
(1975), Kales et al. (1976), and others.

      A common feature of insomniacs is the desire
to avoid stimulation (Coursey et al., 1975;
de la Pena, et al. (1977). In our own lab, we found
that insomniacs consistently report fewer life
changes than normals on the Holmes and Rahe scales.
Coursey et al. (1975) documented that insomniacs
often are sensory reducers. Russian investigators
have postulated that sensory reducing indicates a
"weak nervous system", i.e., excessive arousability
and lability in the ANS.

      According to the formulation by Kales et al.
(1976), insomniacs are characterized by the internalization of psychological disturbances rather
than by acting out. Kales et al. proposed that
this internalization produces a state of constant
emotional arousal which results in generalized
physiological activation and causes the insomnia.

      Excessive ANS arousal is certainly a hallmark
of the insomniac, both during wakefulness and
sleep (Monroe, 1967; Coursey et al., 1975).
Furthermore, poor sleepers take much longer to
reach low levels of activation during sleep than
do good sleepers (Robinson, 1968). However, ANS
arousal is not necessarily the cause of insomnia.
It might be its effect. It will be remembered
that Naitoh et al. (1971b) found a number of conflicting signs of ANS turmoil in their normal,
healthy volunteers after serious, total sleep

deprivation, and that Johnson et al. (1965) found
general ANS arousal following sleep deprivation.

General health also seems to be impaired in
insomniacs. Poor sleepers check
their Cornell Medical Index than good sleepers
(Monroe, 1967). Their general medical malaise
seems to be genuine. Although insomnia is often
explained away as hypochondriasis by the clinician,
both Monroe (1967) and Kales (1976) found that
insomniacs did not score higher than normal on the
MMPI hypochondriasis scale.

Based on the above, sketchy review, it appears
that chronic insomniacs show abundant similarities
to sleep-deprived volunteers in the laboratory.
These similarities include an apparently specific,
dysphoric mood, evidence of ANS arousal, and performance decrements, the latter at least on a
subjective level for the insomniacs. If sleep deprivation caused by such various methods as laboratory stimulation, medical problems, psychopathology,
problems in living, behaviorally bad habits, or
excessive noise, is always followed by a very similar final state, it seems safe to conclude that this
state is caused by sleep deprivation.

Most investigators have usually emphasized
the opposite, i.e., the fact that healthy volunteers
can function quite adequately after a few nights of
sleep deprivation, while the insomniac feels almost
totally incapacitated by just slightly curtailed
sleep. However, this comparison seems unfair because it compares an early deprivation night (no
later than the tenth night) of a healthy volunteer
with what might well be the 1000th night of poor
sleep in the insomniac. Most likely, the insomniacs
have by that time worn down their reserves, while
the volunteers can still draw on them. That this
might be the case has been shown by Williams and
Williams (1966) who found that poor, restless
sleepers reacted much worse to sleep deprivation
than sound sleepers. In addition, volunteers
often look upon the sleepless nights as a challenge,
while insomniacs are panicked by them because they
have so many times associated poor nights with
frustration and difficulties in functioning on the
subsequent day. Furthermore, the volunteers
schedule their sleep deprivation experiments at
a convenient time, while these nights overcome

insomniacs usually at the most inopportune times.

There are, of course, some differences between
experimental sleep deprivation and insomnia, and
they hopefully will help separate the cause from
the results of insomnia. For example, the excessive
psychopathology demonstrated by most insomniacs has
not been recreated in laboratory experiments on
sleep deprivation. This psychopathology is therefore most likely not the result of sleep loss, but
part of its cause. Nevertheless, Webb (1975) describes how sleep deprivation magnifies and potent-
iates pre-existing psychopathologies, and most of
us have probably experienced the fact that our
own weaknesses are harder to control after sleepless nights.

The main problem in trying to learn about the
functions of sleep by studying insomniacs relates
to the cyclicity of the phenomenon. Poor sleep
aggravates psychopathology and causes poor mood and
ANS arousal, which in turn disturb sleep in an end-
less, vicious cycle. It is extremely difficult to
discern whether poor sleep or poor wakefulness
came first. To show that chronic insomnia causes
the waking disturbances seen in insomniacs, one
would need to take good sleepers, healthy both
psychiatrically and medically, and somehow turn
them into chronic insomniacs. This is ethically
not possible.

In my own lab, we are working on the opposite:
we are attempting to change insomniacs into good
sleepers without significantly touching their
psychopathology or their physiological/medical
problems. This is done by various forms of biofeedback. Waking dysphoric mood, psychopathology,
and ANS arousal should improve with sleep improvement to the extent that they are results of poor
sleep. They should remain unchanged by sleep improvement to the extent that they are etiological
factors in insomnia.

In one of our studies, we have treated 30 insomniacs (verified by laboratory sleep) with various forms of biofeedback (frontalis EMG, sensorimotor rhythm, etc.). In 12 patients, such treatment was associated in time with marked improvement of their insomnia. Eleven patients did not learn biofeedback and did not improve their sleep. The remaining cases either did not learn biofeedback but still improved their sleep, or learned biofeedback but did not improve their sleep. They were discarded from this analysis. A control group of 10 insomniacs was tested in the lab, but received no biofeedback.

Each patient slept in the lab twice for three nights each, once at the beginning, and once, a year later, for follow-up. Criteria for improved sleep were based on lab sleep: 10% improvement in sleep efficiency from initial to follow-sleep, more than 30 minutes improvement in sleep latency, or more than 5 spontaneous awakenings less per night.

Figure 1 shows results from the MAACL. Clearly, those insomniacs who improved their sleep through biofeedback felt less "depressed" and less hostile one year later. Based on the discussion above, we would speculate that these feelings initially had been consequences of their poor sleep. On the other hand, improved sleep did not significantly change feelings of anxiety. This would suggest that anxiety mainly was a basic, possibly etiological factor in insomnia, not its consequence. Although these findings sound like common sense, it appears that this is the first time it has been demonstrated that a behavioral, non-psychiatric intervention, if it successfully improves sleep, will chronically improve a person's mood disposition a year later.

What have we learned from this review? Data from sleep deprivation experiments and from work with insomniacs converge and suggest that lack of enough sleep is associated with a specific, dysphoric mood during subsequent wakefulness. If the sleep deprivation is extended, no matter what the etiology, lack of sleep also results in ANS

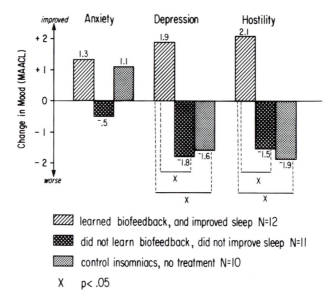

Fig. 1. Change in mood during 1 year in former-
ly chronic insomniacs.

changes, in performance decrements, and in some
neurological impairment. Thus, there is no question that we sleep, at least in part, in order to
function and feel well during subsequent wakefulness. In other words, one function of sleep
is to avoid subsequent deterioration in performance
and mood. What we have not found to date is the
mediator that associates sleep with the subsequent
maintenance of performance and mood.

    Today, the main argument seems to be between
the restorative theory of sleep, and Webb's
adaptive behavioral theory. As Rechtschaffen has
shown during this symposium, this argument cannot
be settled by one conclusive fact or one experiment.

Rather, a network of interacting facts will finally
lead to the gradual acceptance of one theory and to
the gradual rejection of another.

The facts discussed in this paper favor a
restorative theory of sleep. They are, however,
compatible with any one of the five sleep theories
discussed by Webb during this symposium. An
adaptive behavioral theory, for example, might claim
that evolution has so ingrained the sleep-wake
system in the mammalian organism that its disturbance alone causes the general malaise described in
this paper as a result of sleep loss.

Obviously, at this point I personally favor
the restorative theory. Here are my reasons:

1. The wide variability of sleep needs, and
their near perfect adaptation to each animal's life
style is said to favor the adaptive behavioral
theory of sleep. However, to me, this seems to be
weak reasoning. Assume that the concept of calories
had not yet been discovered. One would then be
very impressed by the wide variety of food intakes
in the animal kingdom and by the near perfect adaptation of food intake to the environment: reindeer
thrive best on tundra grasses and burros on thistle;
the tiger eats only a few pounds (of flesh) per
day, but the elephant gulps down nearly half a ton
(of leaves). Where there is much food, grazing
animals eat much, and are larger than those that
live in the near desert and eat less. Using the
arguments of the adaptive behavioral theory, we
might then speculate that there is no restorative
function in eating! Using the same arguments, we
might further conclude that the main function of
eating is adaptational, possible to keep one's
ecological niche free from overcrowding by intrud-
ing animals and plants! Obviously an unlikely theory.

2. All mammals sleep. While this is very
adaptive for most, there are some animals (large
grazing animals without places to hide) for which
no sleep at all would be more adaptive. Reviewing
the animal kingdom, we find that purely adaptive
functions are discarded when they are no longer
useful, while functions that are necessary to life
obviously are not. Vision, for example, is a
purely adaptive function that has been discarded
by mammals that live in permanent darkness. Eating,
on the other hand, is a function necessary for life,
and it has therefore not been discarded by any

single animal species. The fact that all mammals
sleep, even when not sleeping would be more
adaptive for some species, strikes a telling blow
for the restorative theory of sleep.

3. Except for the most primitive mammals,
all show REM and non-REM sleep. For the adaptive
theory of sleep, one state of hypoarousal would
suffice. Where different adaptational solutions
are compatible with survival, different animal
species generally show a wide variety of solutions.
This is true, for example, for locomotion. Where
all mammals use exactly the same solution, it
usually means that there is no other. Thus, it
appears that there probably is some reason for
having REM and NREM sleep, and I believe that the
experiments on selective sleep stage deprivation
have already given a glimpse of that reason.

4. The results of sleep deprivation, either
experimental or in clinical insomnia, lean toward
a restorative function of sleep. So does common
sense. While I am quite willing to forego common
sense if the facts show otherwise, in my judgement this has not yet been done by the proponents
of the adaptive theory.

5. Proponents of the adaptive theory often
claim that, if restoration were accomplished during
sleep, the organism would sustain more damage from
sleepless nights, and not just feel poorly. Permit
me a speculative note. How do we force animals or
people to behave according to our own wishes? We
make them feel poorly when they do not, feel well
when they do what we desire. Assume that sleep,
for whatever reason, is important for the survival
of the organism, but that it is also important that
during emergencies the organisms be able to perform
without sleep. I can think of no more efficient
mechanism to keep an organism on the routine sleep-
wake schedule than to disturb its mood if it does
not sleep. This is a very unpleasant, but nevertheless not crucial aspect of functioning. Then,
if that sign is not heeded, the organism gets
further prodded into sleep by more insistent, but
still non-life-threatening signs, such as hand
tremors, difficulties in eye focusing, and ANS
disturbances. In other words, while the function
of sleep is still debatable, we seem to be so
constructed that we are invariable prodded into

sleeping by the most gentle, but nevertheless
almost totally effective means that are available
in nature. This is, of course, what Webb meant
when he called sleep "the gentle tyrant".
    In sum, the argument is not settled, but in
my judgement, the data lean towards sleep having
some kind of restorative function.

REFERENCES

Agnew, H. W., Jr., Webb, W. B., Williams, R. L.
    Comparison of stage four and 1-REM sleep
    deprivation. Perceptual and Motor Skills, 24:
    851-858, 1967.

Cartwright, R. D. Night Life, Explorations in
    Dreaming. Englewood Cliffs, N. J.: Prentice-
    Hall, 1977.

Coursey, R. D., Buchsbaum, M., and Frankel, B. L.
    Personality measures and evoked responses in
    chronic insomniacs. Journal of Abnormal
    Psychology, 84: 239-249, 1975.

de la Pena, A., Flickinger, R., and Mayfield, D.
    Reverse first-night effect in chronic poor
    sleepers. In Chase, M.M., Mitler, M.M., and
    Walters, P.L. (Eds.), Sleep Research, v. 6, Los
    Angeles, BIS/BRI, 1977, p. 167

Dement, W. C. Sleep deprivation and the organiza-
    tion of the behavioral states. In E. D.
    Clemente, D. P. Purpura, and F. E. Mayer (Eds.),
    Sleep and the Maturing Nervous System. New
    York: Academic Press, 1972, pp. 319-361.

Fischer-Perroudon, C., Mouret, J., and Jouvet, M.
    Sur un cas d'agrypnie (4 mois sans sommeil)
    au cours d'une maladie de morvan. Effet
    favorable du 5-hydroxytryptophane. Electro-
    encephalography and Clinical Neurophysiology,
    36: 1-18, 1974.

Globus, G. G. A syndrome associated with sleeping
    late. Psychosomatic Medicine, 31: 528-535,
    1969.

Hartmann, E. L.   The Functions of Sleep.   New Haven:
     Yale University Press, 1973.

Hartmann, E., Baekeland, F., and Zwilling, G. R.
     Psychological differences between long and
     short sleepers. Archives of General Psychiatry,
     26: 463-468, 1972.

Hauri, P.   Effects of evening activity on subsequent
     sleep and dreams. Unpublished doctoral disser-
     tation, University of Chicago, 1966.

Hauri, P.   Insomnia and other sleep disorders.   In
     F. Kagan et al. (Eds.), Hypnotics: Methods of
     Development and Evaluation. New York:
     Spectrum Publications, 1975.

Hauri, P.   A case series analysis of 141 consecutive
     insomniacs evaluated at the Dartmouth Sleep
     Lab.   In M. H. Chase, M. M. Mitler, P. L.
     Walter (Eds.), Sleep Research, Volume 5.   Los
     Angeles: Brain Information Service/Brain
     Research Institute, 1976, p. 173.

Johnson, L. C.   Are stages of sleep related to
     waking behavior? American Scientist, 61: 326-
     338, 1973.

Johnson, L. C. and MacLeod, W. L.   Sleep and awake
     behavior during gradual sleep reduction.
     Perceptual and Motor Skills, 36: 87-97, 1973.

Johnson, L. C., Slye, E. S., and Dement, W.
     Electroencephalographic and autonomic activity
     during and after prolonged sleep deprivation.
     Psychosomatic Medicine, 27: 415-423, 1965.

Kales, A., Caldwell, A. B., Preston, T. A., Healey,
     S., Kales, J. D.   Personality patterns in
     insomnia. Archives of General Psychiatry, 33:
     1128-1134, 1976.

Kales, A. and Kales, J. D.   Sleep disorders:
     recent findings in the diagnosis and treatment
     of disturbed sleep. New England Journal of
     Medicine, 290: 487-499, 1974.

Karacan, I., Williams, R. L., Littell, R. C., and
    Salis, P. J. Insomniacs: unpredictable and
    idiosyncratic sleepers. In W. P. Koella
    and P. Levin (Eds.), Sleep. Basel: S. Karger,
    1973, pp. 120-132.

Kollar, E. J., Namerow, N., Pasnau, R. O., and
    Naitoh, P. Neurological findings during
    prolonged sleep deprivation. Neurology, 18:
    836-840, 1968.

Moldofsky, H. and Scarisbrick, P. Induction of
    neurasthenic musculoskeletal pain syndrome
    by selective sleep stage deprivation. Psycho-
    somatic Medicine, 38: 35-44, 1976.

Monroe, L. J. Psychological and physiological
    differences between good and poor sleepers.
    Journal of Abnormal Psychology, 72: 255-264,
    1967.

Naitoh, P., Johnson, L. C., and Lubin, A. Modifi-
    cation of surface negative slow potential
    (CNV) in the human brain after total sleep
    loss. Electroencephalography and Clinical
    Neurophysiology, 30: 17-22, 1971 a.

Naitoh, P., Pasnau, R. O., and Kollar, E. J.
    Psychophysiological changes after prolonged
    deprivation of sleep. Biological Psychiatry,
    3: 309-320, 1971 b.

Pasnau, R. O., Naitoh, P., Stier, S., and Kollar,
    E. J. The psychological effects of 205 hours
    of sleep deprivation. Archives of General
    Psychiatry, 18: 496-505, 1968.

Robinson, T. M. Presleep activity and sleep quali-
    ty in good and poor sleepers. Unpublished
    doctoral dissertation, University of Chicago,
    1969.

Ross, J. J. Neurological findings after prolonged
    sleep deprivation. Archives of Neurology,
    12: 399-403, 1965.

Stuss, D., Healey, T., and Broughton, R. Personali-
ty and performance measures in natural extreme
short sleepers. In M. H. Chase, W. C. Stern,
P. L Walter (Eds.), Sleep Research, Volume 4.
Los Angeles: Brain Information Service/Brain
Research Institute, 1975, p. 204.

Taub, J. M. and Berger, R. J. The effects of
changing the phase and duration of sleep.
Journal of Experimental Psychology: Human
Perception and Performance, 2: 30-41, 1976.

Taub, J. M., Globus, G. G., Phoebus, E., Drury, R.
Extended sleep and performance. Nature, 233:
142-143, 1971.

Townsend, R. E., Prinz, P. N., Obrist, W. D.
Human cerebral blood flow during sleep and
waking. Journal of Applied Physiology, 35:
620-625, 1973.

Vogel, G. W., Thurmond, A., Gibbons, P., Sloan, K.,
Boyd, M., and Walker, M. REM sleep reduction
effects on depression syndromes. Archives of
General Psychiatry, 32: 765-777, 1975.

Wagner, M. K. and Mooney, D. K. Personality
characteristics of long and short sleepers.
Journal of Clinical Psychology, 31: 434-436,
1975.

Walter, W. G., Cooper, R., Aldridge, V. J.,
McCallum, W. G., and Winter, A. L. Contingent
negative variation: an electric sign of
sensorimotor association and expectancy in
the human brain. Nature, 203: 380-384, 1964.

Webb, W. B. Sleep, the Gentle Tyrant. Englewood
Cliffs, N. J.: Prentice-Hall, 1975.

Webb, W. B. and Friel, J. Sleep stage and personality characteristics of "natural" long and
short sleepers. Science, 171: 587-588, 1971.

Wilkinson, R. T., Edwards, R. S., and Haines, E.
Performance following a night of reduced
sleep. Psychonomic Science, 5: 471-472, 1966.

Williams, R. L. and Karacan, I. Sleep disorders and disordered sleep. In M. F. Reiser (Ed.), Organic Disorders and Psychosomatic Medicine (Volume 4 of American Handbook of Psychiatry). New York: Basic Books, 1975, pp. 854-904.

Williams, H. L. and Williams, C. L. Nocturnal EEG profiles and performance. Psychophysiology, 3: 164-175, 1966.

Zarcone, V., de la Pena, A., and Dement, W. C. Heightened sexual interest and sleep disturbance. Perceptual and Motor Skills, 39: 1135-1141, 1974.

THE RELEVANCE OF SLEEP PATHOLOGIES
TO THE FUNCTION OF SLEEP

WILLIAM C. DEMENT

Sleep Research Center
Stanford University School of Medicine
Stanford, California

Introduction

The function of sleep heads the list of the very important issues in sleep research today. It is one of the great mysteries that, as Albert Einstein said, are the sources of all art and science. In recent years, the description and treatment of specific sleep pathologies has become available as a new resource in the search for function. My presentation will highlight a few of these clinical findings with the air of examining their relevance to the question of sleep function. In addition, I will present a new approach to the problems of sleepiness that we are developing at Stanford.

Sleep Pathologies

This symposium coincides with the publication of a new book, The Sleep Instinct, by Ray Meddis (1977) which presents detailed arguments for a point of view that was heralded by Webb in 1971 and is very relevant to the present discussion. In essence, Meddis regards sleep and all of the related behavior as an instinct that served an important purpose early in man's history--that of promoting energy conservation and security--but a purpose that is not necessary in modern society. Thus, if there could be an atraumatic enucleation of a center controlling the sleep instinct, we would be none the worse and, indeed, except for potential boredom, might be much better. From the viewpoint of a sleep clinician, if indeed sleep or the adaptive advantage it entails is not necessary, if man could live just as well without sleep, then we should move as

273

Copyright © 1979 by Academic Press, Inc.
All rights of reproduction in any form reserved.
ISBN 0-12-222340-3

quickly as possible to rid ourselves of it. For
it is becoming more and more evident that in many
ways sleep is a curse, not a blessing. We now
know, for example, that it is possible for human
beings to die during sleep even though they appear
to be, and probably are, completely healthy when
awake. Halberg et al. (1976) have recently called
attention to the fact that the overall death rate
for humans is considerably higher at night than
during the daytime.

One of the most clear-cut examples of a
specific high risk sleep pathology are the group
of sleep apnea syndromes (Guilleminault et al.,
1976, Guilleminault and Dement, 1978). This group
of illnesses involves serious respiratory disturbances that exist exclusively during sleep. Although
longitudinal data are very sparse, it is likely
that these syndromes are terminal illnesses. The
consequences of the illness can include serious
hemodynamic abnormalities, sleep related cardio-
rhythmic abnormalities, profound daytime hyper-
somnolence, and finally, the specter of sudden
unexpected death during sleep. Thus, individuals
who suffer from sleep apnea would certainly be far
better off if they did not sleep at all. Yet
Meddis (1977) makes a great point that the evolution of sleep was favored because sleep was
advantageous to the organism. What he failed to
consider was that, at least in terms of respiratory
function and associated cardiac function, sleep
can also put the organism in a state of high risk.
Figure 1 shows an example of a sleep apnea associated cardiac arrhythmia in a patient, which is
seen only during sleep and doubtless explains why
some sleep apnea patients die suddenly in their
sleep.

Short of a full-blown upper airway sleep
apnea syndrome, it appears that sleep increases
everyone's risk in terms of an increase in airway
resistance. Orem et al. (1977) have demonstrated
in cats substantial overall increases in airway
resistance that are exquisitely related to the
occurrence of sleep. Figure 2 shows a polygraph
tracing that can serve as an example of the preci-
sion of this relationship. Orem (1977) has recently reported that these changes seem to involve a
sleep-related failure of the CNS coordination of
breathing and the activity of the laryngeal muscles.

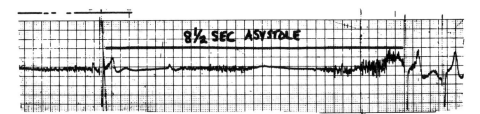

Fig. 1. Electrocardiogram tracing from a patient during one of his repetitive episodes of sleep apnea. The tracing shows an unusually prolonged asystole.

In humans, a ubiquitous increase in airway resistance during sleep is dramatically demonstrated by snoring. With a pressure transducer in the thoracic esophagus, we have shown that the same airflow as prior wakefulness is associated with a five-fold greater amplitude of endoesophageal pressure changes during snoring. There is virtually no change in amplitude when a non-snorer falls asleep. Various surveys (Boulware, 1974; Lugaresi et al., 1978) suggest that about 50 percent of all adult males and 30 percent of adult females snore. These findings have implications beyond the prima facie evidence of increased airway resistance. In 1975, Lugaresi and his colleagues studied eight normal males whose only problem was a history of heavy snoring. This study clearly showed the relationship among snoring, increased airway resistance, and sleep apnea by documenting upper airway apneas and hemodynamic abnormalities during sleep in all eight subjects. So we ask ourselves--why didn't evolution (or Mother Nature) provide for better airway function during sleep?

We have long assumed that regulatory processes, particularly those involving peripheral feedback loops and brain stem circuitry, are essentially the same during quiet wakefulness and sleep. In other words, we assume that in both wakefulness and sleep, CO_2 levels provoke a respiratory drive and Hering-Breuer reflexes provide a major

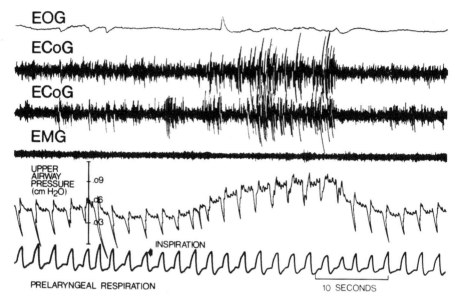

Fig. 2.   Relationship between level of
arousal and upper airway resistance in the cat.
Note that as sleep develops there is an increase
in upper airway resistance and that there is a
decrease beginning simultaneously with the electro-
cortical arousal.   This second by second relationship is typical.   When sleep is maintained, the
increase in resistance will also be maintained.
EOG: electro-oculogram; ECoG: electrocorticogram;
EMG: electromyographic activity from nuchal muscles.
(After Orem et al., 1977).

organizing input for the cyclic alternation of
inspiration and expiration.   This is absolutely
wrong.   These regulatory mechanisms are greatly
altered by sleep.   Indeed, a certain amount of
evidence is accumulating to suggest that an entirely separate respiratory mechanism may obtain during
sleep. Phillipson et al. (1977) have elegantly
demonstrated in the dog, as was mentioned earlier,
that one of the most crucial elements subserving
respiratory regulation during wakefulness (CO_2
response) does not play a role in REM sleep.

Phillipson et al. (1976) have also demonstrated
that the absence of vagal input does not affect
breathing in REM sleep. Thus, we might imagine,
as Phillipson and Sullivan (1978) propose, that
there is an entirely different program or neurological sunstrate for breathing in REM sleep.

The existence of such a separate neurological
substrate for breathing during REM sleep is a
possibility supported by the findings of Netick
et al. (1977) in the cat. These findings included
the presence of units in the brain stem respiratory
areas that fire only in REM sleep and whose overall
rate of firing is related to the rate of respiration. These units may in effect substitute for
the "wakefulness stimulus," the absence of which
was proposed by Fink et al. (1963) to account for
the sleep-related hypocarbic apnea response.

There is other evidence, particularly related
to REM sleep, suggesting dramatically different
regulatory programs in functions other than respiration. For example, Glotzbach and Heller (1976)
have gathered evidence that temperature regulation
ceases in REM sleep. The well-known tonic motor
inhibition in REM sleep also suggests altered
neural programming. Finally, there also appear to
be cardiac abnormalities that are sleep induced,
as evidenced by our findings in certain infants
(who were nearmiss for sudden infant death
syndrome)[1] of profound bradycardia that appeared
frequently in sleep but never in the waking state
(Guilleminault and Ariagno, in preparation). We
have also seen several patients in our Sleep
Disorders Center at Stanford who showed very
prolonged asystoles during sleep although respiration appeared to be entirely normal. One case was
so severe that a cardiac pacemaker was implanted.

In 1971, Allan Rechtschaffen made the following observation in a discussion of the purpose of
sleep: "If sleep does not serve an absolutely
vital function, then it is the biggest mistake the
evolutionary process ever made." Rechtschaffen
went on to point out that sleep precludes hunting
for and consuming food; it is also incompatible
with procreation. Although Rechtschaffen's
concerns have been addressed by Meddis (1977),
neither Rechtschaffen nor anyone else in 1971 per-
ceived the astonishing magnitude of the evolutionary mistake that sleep might be. To the extent

that sleep is incompatible with normal respiratory
function, for example, can sleep be considered a
viable adaptive response? Or, are we continuing
to miss something that is so important that its
needs must be served even though the price, as we
have seen is rather high?

Sleepiness and the Function of Sleep

Putting aside for the moment the question of
nature's fallibility, after centuries of taking it
for granted, why do we now doubt that sleep serves
a vital purpose? Much of our doubt arises from
the many studies that have failed to show any
change in the sleep deprived organism that could
implicate a vital function. For the Stanford group,
the watershed was the 264-hour wakefulness marathon
of Randy Gardner (Gulevich et al., 1966), who
failed to exhibit any dramatic functional impairment during the procedure. Studies of blood and
urine during sleep and sleep loss have not demonstrated a vital restorative function. In the case
of REM sleep, it has been apparently extirpated
for a year or more with no obvious ill effects
(Wyatt et al., 1971). Behavioral impairments
that accompany sleep loss, such as performance
decrements, have been attributed to increasing
neuromuscular fatigue. Yet this "fatigue" has
not been clearly demonstrated, and it is becoming
clear that such performance changes are really due
to drowsiness (Guilleminault et al., 1975). Thus
we have become convinced that the major consequence
of sleep loss is sleepiness; and it is remarkable
that sleepiness has received so little study.[2] As
Meddis (1977) notes, "It is a pity that the recent
intensive sleep research effort has almost totally
ignored the magical phenomenon of drowsiness" (p.8).
Even though sleepiness is an attribute of the
awake individual and independent of sleep per se,
as the most reliable consequence of sleep loss it
ought to be an important concern of sleep research.
There is, however, no established tradition of
investigative approaches except indirectly through
performance testing; and there are certainly no
widely accepted definitions nor a sizeable body
of knowledge. We have been investigating sleepiness, more or less directly, for the past five

years and have adopted two axioms as fundamental
to this work. The first is that sleepiness is an
elemental feeling state that is accessible to
introspection and discriminable from related
feeling states such as physical <u>fatigue</u>, <u>depression</u>,
and other dysphorias. The second axiom is that
sleepiness is essentially a physiological drive
state (or instinct) that occurs in response to
sleep loss and leads to sleep-seeking behavior,
as well as an increased tendency to fall asleep
(Dement, 1976).

Our first attempts to deal more systematically
with this dimension led to the development of the
<u>Stanford Sleepiness Scale (SSS)</u>, a 7-point, Likert
self-rating scale (Hoddes et al., 1972), and the
cross-validation of the SSS with measures of performance before, during and after sleep deprivation
(Hoddes et al., 1973). The Stanford Sleepiness
Scale is reproduced in Table I. Although the SSS
has been a useful tool, particularly in ease and
cheapness of administration, it has proven to have
an important disadvantage in its overall consist-
ency.

Accordingly, we have attempted to move to a
more objective and quantitative measure of sleep
tendency. Because the exact time of transition
from wakefulness to sleep is relatively easy to
specify in polygraphic recordings (figure 3), it
has been possible to design a standard situation
in which the momentary sleep tendency of an individual can be measured by the speed of falling
asleep, or sleep latency. Thus we have come to
use repeated determinations of sleep latency as a
measure of sleep tendency and have validated this
measurement using the most predictable cause of
subjective sleepiness--total sleep deprivation.

In a study by Carskadon and Dement (in press),
six normal college students (4 men, 2 women) aged
18-20 years were observed before, during, and after
total sleep loss. Every two hours during the time
they were awake and out of bed, a sleep latency
test (SLT) was administered. For each test the
subjects went to bed in individual rooms and were
instructed to close their eyes, lie quietly, and
try to fall asleep. The beginning of measurement
was the exact moment of "lights out," and the test
was terminated after one minute of sleep.

TABLE I

STANFORD SLEEPINESS SCALE

Code

1 **Feeling active and vital; alert; wide awake**
2 **Functioning at a high level; but not at peak; able to concentrate**
3 **Relaxed; awake; not at full alertness; responsive**
4 **A little foggy, not at peak; let down**
5 **Fogginess, beginning to lose interest in remaining awake; slowed down**
6 **Sleepiness; prefer to be lying down; fighting sleep, woozy**
7 **Almost in reverie, sleep onset soon; lost struggle to remain awake**
X **Asleep** (If you are sleeping during any of the time periods, then write "X" for these periods)

	0-15	15-30	30-45	45-60	Comments
Midnight 0000					
0100					
0200					
0300					
0400					
0500					
0600					
0700					
0800					
0900					
1000					
1100					
Noon 1200					
1300					
1400					
1500					
1600					
1700					
1800					
1900					
2000					
2100					
2200					
2300					

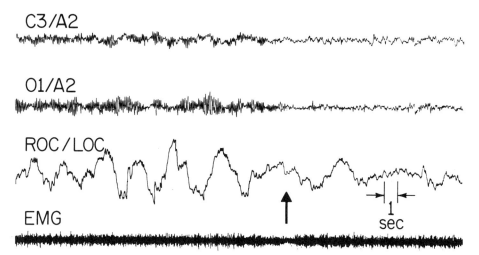

Fig. 3. Polygraphic tracing of sleep onset. The upper channels are taken from monopolar recordings of central and occipital electroencephalogram. The third tracing is a recording of eye movements from left and right outer canthi using electrooculogram. The bottom tracing is a bipolar surface electromyogram from the chin. Sleep onset occurs at the arrow, which represents a change from relaxed wakefulness (note alpha rhythm in EEG channels) to stage 1 NREM sleep. The tracings were made at a paper speed of 10 mm/sec.

If subjects remained awake by EEG criteria, the sleep latency test was terminated after 20 minutes. The sleep latency score was judged as the interval in half minutes between the start of the test and first 30-second epoch scored as NREM stage 1 sleep. These procedures prevented the accumulation of substantial quantities of sleep.

As Figure 4 illustrates, the results were dramatic. In all subjects sleep latency declined in the middle of the first night to minimum levels (less than one minute) that were maintained until sleep was permitted. SLT scores returned to baseline values only after the second recovery night. The most striking departure from conventional

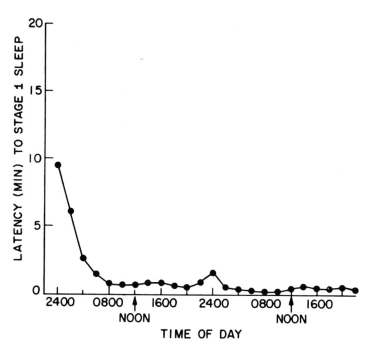

Fig. 4. (A) Sleep latencies during total sleep deprivation. Graph begins at 2400 on the first night without sleep. Sleep latency is measured every 2 hours during the period of enforced wakefulness. Each point represents the mean value for 6 subjects. Note the almost immediate decrease in sleep latency to less than one minute, a value which is maintained essentially unchanged for the remainder of the vigil.

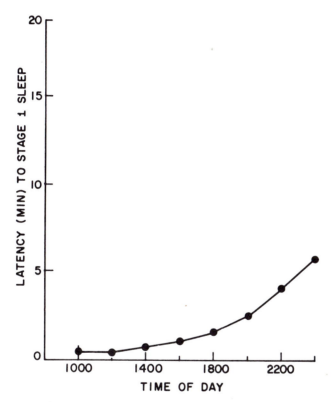

Fig. 4. (B) Sleep latencies throughout the day following the first night of recovery sleep. The first test of the day at 1000 is at the same level as the final tests during sleep deprivation. Apparently no recovery in sleep latency has taken place. Remarkably, sleepiness decreases during wakefulness.

rationales about sleep loss were the sleep latency
scores on the first day following an entire night
of sleep. Early on the first recovery day, the
sleep latencies were very short and only gradually
through the day returned to basal levels.

Several questions of interest arise from these
findings. First, the maximum consequence of sleep
loss--that is, virtually instantaneous sleep onset
whenever sleep was permitted--occurred almost immediately. The subjects reached this level within
several hours after sleep loss began, and thus were
maximally sleepy, although indexes of performance
were only marginally affected at the time. Thus,
it appeared that maximum sleepiness occurred almost
as an all or none response. This finding is in
conflict with the notion of a slow deterioration.
In addition, the sleepiness response was not completely reversed by a full night of sleep, as has
been found with performance decrements. It would
be of interest, however, to see what would happen
if longer amounts of recovery sleep were allowed.
Finally, it is not clear whether the sleepiness
response resulted from sleep loss itself or was a
function of normal circadian change.

The mention of circadian factors brings to
mind another validation of the SLT procedure--the
90-minute day studies (Carskadon and Dement, 1975;
1977). Ten college students, aged 17-21,
volunteered to go to bed every 90 minutes around
the clock, staying in bed 30 minutes each time.
This schedulre represented a slight variation of
the foregoing study in that the sleep periods were
not terminated immediately after sleep onset and
sleep could accumulate over 24 hours up to 30
minutes on each test. This procedure was designed
to obviate the extreme sleepiness of total sleep
loss and to allow a circadian rhythm of sleepiness
and alertness to manifest itself independent of
clock time. Figure 5 shows in a typical subject
that pronounced circadian fluctuations in sleep
latency scores appeared over the five days of the
study. Parenthetically, the shortest latencies
did not occur during conventional sleeping hours,
which may be a peculiarity of college students.

It should be emphasized that ordinarily,
sleep deprivation studies are highly structured
situations in which subjects going without sleep

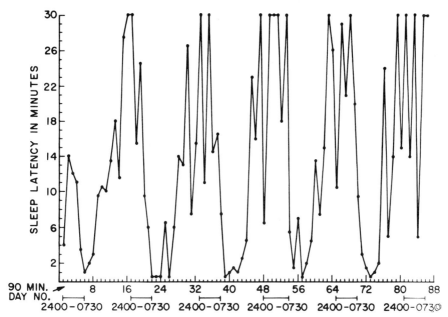

Fig. 5. Eighty-six consecutive sleep latency tests in one typical subject. Results are not pooled because individual differences in peak-trough timing would obscure the clear circadian rhythm of sleepiness. In this study, sleep latency was measured every 90 minutes (16 times a day). The intermittent bars under the abscissa show the conventional bedtime hours. Most subjects did not experience their greatest sleepiness during these hours as can be seen in the graph.

receive an incredible amount of support to offset the sleep tendency. It would be impossible for anyone to remain awake continuously for any length of time in the face of maximum sleepiness without such massive assistance. Therefore, because of the paradoxical motivation in such situations, there is a tendency to avoid dwelling on the misery of extreme sleepiness. It is clear, however, that

subjects can endure the discomfort only because
they can look forward to the ultimate relief.
Further, it is possible that once sleepiness is
maximal, the continued effort to fight it off and
to maintain wakefulness is only a stress over and
above the sleepiness response--a stress that can
only confound the situation.

At this point it is of interest to elaborate
a general consideration of sleep deprivation
studies, as well as the observations of Meddis et
al. (1973) and Jones and Oswald (1968) on nonsleepers. An issue that is of no little interest
is that, in essence, total sleep loss is virtually
impossible to maintain without second-by-second
EEG monitoring and a way to prevent the development of sleep. The increasing tendency to sleep
seems eventually to reach an equilibrium in which
intense pressure for sleep is maintained at a
steady state by multiple microsleep episodes. In
fact, 100% wakefulness has not been demonstrated
in any study of sleep loss. The problem with REM
sleep deprivation is somewhat more complicated
because REM sleep can dissociate into two or more
components that are difficult to identify in iso-
lation. Thus we cannot assume that the perfect
sleep or REM sleep deprivation study has actually
been done.

In terms of total sleep loss, it is important
to determine whether the sleepiness response that
we have described in humans is nothing more than
a reflection of a circadian oscillation of sleep
tendency that obtains when there is an unexpected
interruption of the events that ordinarily drive
or program the reversal of the circadian sleepiness
curve. Extreme partial sleep deprivation might
shed some light on this question, as in the studies
of Johnson and MacLeod (1973). Although subjects
in this study complained of sleepiness and gave
it as their major reason for terminating, sleepiness
was not measured objectively. Thus, they could
just have been very bored. A recent study at
Stanford of partial sleep loss in children, reducing
the allotment from 10 to 4 hours on a single night,
showed a marked, though not maximal increase of
sleepiness (Carskadon et al., in press). There
is also a need to investigate with objective
measures the sleepiness or sleep tendency of the

so-called nonsleepers or short sleepers, although
from my personal interactions with such individuals,
I must say that they did not appear to be at all
sleepy.

  To return to a consideration of sleep pathologies, what are our expectations with regard to
their sleepiness response? If we take the pathology of narcolepsy in which the chief complaint
is extreme sleepiness, we might ask whether we
will see the same sort of sleep tendency profile
that was found in normal subjects after sleep loss.
Figure 6, illustrating the results of multiple
sleep latency tests in a group of narcoleptic
patients, suggests that the pattern is the same.

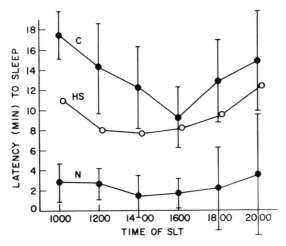

  Fig. 6. Multiple sleep latency tests in
eight patients with narcolepsy (N). Note that the
patients are much sleepier than the comparison
groups (HS, C). Vertical bars represent one
standard deviation.

  Continuing to assume that sleepiness is a
state that occurs in response to sleep loss, we
might conclude that patients with narcolepsy are

are somehow locked into this state. No matter
how much sleep they experience each day, they do
not switch to the alert state. We have previously
suggested that if there were some way to make the
fight worth while, a person could fight off the
urge to sleep and endure total sleep loss more or
less indefinitely. If the patient with narcolepsy
is analogous to a totally sleep deprived person,
we can conclude that the major consequence of sleep
loss, namely sleepiness, is not in and of itself
harmful. As far as we know, narcolepsy does not
carry any implication of shortening life span or
undermining physical health. On the other hand,
to be sleepy all the time is very close to being
dead in the opinion of many patients. Therefore,
if the sole function of sleep in the normal individual is to prevent extreme sleepiness, it is a
sufficient justification.

What about insomnia, most prevalent of all
sleep disorder complaints? We would have been
surprised that insomniacs do not complain of
sleepiness during the day, except that we have
found that these patients are not sleep deprived
in the usual sense of the word. In fact, many
patients who complain of insomnia appear to obtain
a considerable amount of sleep (Carskadon et al.,
1976). In extreme cases, the urgency of the
insomnia complaint leads us to wonder if there is
not an abnormality of the sleepiness response so
that instead of getting sleepy, the patients
experience some other change, such as depression
or anxiety. This would allow us to posit chronic
anxiety as a cause of insomnia, if we assume that
the anxiety is somehow substituting for the sleepiness response, which in a normal individual would
limit the insomnia by increasing sleep tendency.
It is my belief, however, that there is no amount
of anxiety that can override the sleepiness response indefinitely. This was recently demonstrated
by Dr. Heinz Tanberg, a psychoanalyst (personal
communication) who found that by keeping a group
of severely phobic patients awake all night, the
phobias were at least temporarily relieved by
substituting one complaint (sleepiness) for another.

Concluding Remarks

The formal study of sleep pathologies as a clinical discipline is just beginning. However, we have already achieved new insights into the complexity of the states of sleep. Even one small part of this complexity, the control of respiration as a function of state, could be called an exciting new frontier in medicine with enormous implications for health and disease. Sleep in its totality and imbedded in the circadian cycle and the life cycle is overwhelming. Even so, theories of the function of sleep must take all of the data into account. There is a great need for formalism in the field of sleep research to make sure that researchers are aware of all the pertinent data and do not waste time with inadequate tests of inadequately formulated hypotheses.

My final comment is that I sometimes feel we have placed too great a reliance on reasoning from the principles of natural selection and adaptive evolution. To underscore this point and to end this essay on a lighter note, I will mention a very private and personal theory of REM sleep. Is it possible that REM sleep exists not because of the evolutionary past, but because it is part of some cosmic program to prepare man for an interstellar future? Havelock Ellis once said, "A dream is real while it lasts. Can we say more of life?" Can the dream reality enable us, should we learn to use it more efficiently, to test alternate realities or to experience and plan for totally new realities? I have a certain affinity for this viewpoint because of a dream that may have saved my life. Some years ago I was smoking three packs of cigarettes a day. I coughed up blood. I had an X-ray, my lungs were full of cancer, I felt poignantly the intense reality of the premature termination of my life, and then I woke up. Given the opportunity to experience this alternative, the choice was obvious. I have not smoked a cigarette in the intervening 13 years.

FOOTNOTES

[1]More than <u>10,000 infants yearly</u> in the United
States are victims of the sudden infant death
syndrome (<u>SIDS</u>). While the specific cause or
causes remain unknown, the deaths occur in relation to sleep, and many investigators feel that
<u>sleep apnea</u> is one of the most likely possibilities.

[2]Most of the major books dealing with sleep
research, e.g., <u>The Sleeping Brain</u> edited by Chase
(1972), or <u>Sleep and Wakefulness</u> by Kleitman
(1963), do not index "sleepiness" or discuss it
explicitly in the text.

ACKNOWLEDGMENT

Supported by National Institute of Mental
Health Research Scientist Award MH 05804.

REFERENCES

Boulware, M. <u>Snoring</u>. Rockaway, New Jersey:
    American Faculty Press, 1974.

Carskadon, M. and Dement, W. C. Sleep studies on
    a 90-minute day. <u>Electroencephalography</u> and
    <u>Clinical Neurophysiology</u>, <u>39</u>: 145-155, 1975.

Carskadon, M. and Dement, W. C. Sleepiness and
    sleep state on a 90-minute schedule. <u>Psycho-</u>
    <u>physiology</u>, <u>14</u>: 127-133, 1977.

Carskadon, M. and Dement, W. C. Sleep tendency:
    an objective measure of sleep loss. <u>Sleep</u>
    <u>Research</u>, <u>6</u>: 200, 1977.

Carskadon, M., Dement, W. C., Mitler, M.,
    Guilleminault, C., Zarcone, V. and Spiegel, R.
    Self-reports versus sleep laboratory findings
    in 122 drug-free subjects complaining of
    chronic insomnia. <u>American Journal of</u>
    <u>Psychiatry</u>, <u>133</u>: 1382-1388, 1976.

Carskadon, M., Harvey, K., Dement, W. and Anders, T. Acute partial sleep deprivation in children. Sleep Research, 6: 92, 1977.

Chase, M. (Ed.) The Sleeping Brain, Perspectives in the Brain Sciences, Vol. 1. Los Angeles: Brain Information Service, Brain Research Institute, 1972.

Dement, W. Daytime sleepiness and sleep "attacks". In C. Guilleminault, W. Dement, and P. Passouant (Eds.), Narcolepsy. New York: Spectrum Publications, 1976, pp. 17-42.

Fink, B. R., Hanks, E., Hgai, S., and Papper, E. Central regulation of respiration during anesthesia and wakefulness. Annals of the New York Academy of Science 109: 892-900, 1963.

Glotzbach, S. and Heller, C. Central nervous regulation of body temperature during sleep. Science, 194: 537-539, 1976.

Guilleminault, C. and Ariagno, R. Why should we study the infant "near miss for sudden infant death"?, in preparation.

Guilleminault, C. and Dement, W. C. (Eds.) The Sleep Apnea Syndromes. New York: Alan R. Liss, Inc., 1978.

Guilleminault, C., Phillips, R., and Dement, W. C. A syndrome of hypersomnia with automatic behavior. Electroencephalography and Clinical Neurophysiology, 38: 403-413, 1975.

Guilleminault, C., Tilkian, A., and Dement, W. C. The sleep apnea syndromes. Annual Review of Medicine, 27: 465-484, 1976.

Gulevich, G., Dement, W., and Johnson, L. Psychiatric and EEG observations on a case of prolonged (264 hours) wakefulness. Archives General of Psychiatry, 15: 29-35, 1966.

Halberg, F., Louro, R., and Carandente, F. Autorhythmometry. Richerche Clinica di Laboratorio, 6: 207-250, 1976.

Hoddes, E., Dement, W., and Zarcone, V. The development and use of the Stanford Sleepiness Scale (SSS). Psychophysiology, 9: 150, 1972.

Hoddes, E., Zarcone, V., Smythe, H., Phillips, R., and Dement, W. Quantification of sleepiness: a new approach. Psychophysiology, 10: 431-436, 1973.

Johnson, L. and MacLeod, W. Sleep and awake behavior during gradual sleep reduction. Perceptual and Motor Skills, 36: 87-97, 1973.

Jones, H. and Oswald, I. Two cases of healthy insomnia. Electroencephalography and Clinical Neurophysiology, 24: 378-380, 1968.

Kleitman, N. Sleep and Wakefulness. Chicago: University of Chicago Press, 1963.

Lugaresi, E., Coccagna, G., and Cirignotta, F. Snoring and its clinical implications. In C. Guilleminault and W. Dement (Eds.), The Sleep Apnea Syndromes. New York: Alan R. Liss, Inc., 1978.

Lugaresi, E., Coccagna, G., Farneti, P., Mantovani, M. and Cirignotta, F. Snoring. Electroencephalography and Clinical Neurophysiology, 39: 59-64, 1975.

Meddis, R. The Sleep Instinct. London: Routledge and Kegan Paul, 1977.

Meddis, R., Pearson, A., and Langford, G. An extreme case of healthy insomnia. Electroencephalography and Clinical Neurophysiology, 35: 213-214, 1973.

Netick, A., Orem, J. and Dement, W. Neuronal activity specific to REM sleep and its relationship to breathing. Brain Research, 120: 197-207, 1977.

Orem, J. Laryngeal activity during sleep. Sleep Research, 6: 55, 1977.

Orem, J., Netick, A., and Dement, W. Increased upper airway resistance to breathing during sleep in the cat. Electroencephalography and Clinical Neurophysiology, 93: 14-22, 1977.

Phillipson, E., Kozar, L., Rebuck, A., and Murphy, E. Ventilatory and waking responses to CO_2 in sleeping dogs. American Review of Respiratory Diseases, 115: 251-262, 1977.

Phillipson, E., Murphy, E., and Kozar, L. Regulation of respiration in sleeping dogs. Journal of Applied Physiology, 40: 688-694, 1976.

Phillipson, E. and Sullivan, C. Respiratory control mechanisms during non-REM and REM sleep. In C. Guilleminault and W. Dement (Eds.), The Sleep Apnea Syndromes. New York: Alan R. Liss, Inc., 1978.

Rechtschaffen, A. The control of sleep. In W. Hunt (Ed.), Human Behavior and Its Control. Cambridge: Schenkman Publishing Company Inc., 1971.

Webb, W. Sleep as a biorhythm. In P. Colquhoun (Ed.), Biological Rhythms and Human Performance. London: Academic Press, 1971.

Wyatt, R., Fram, D., Buchbinder, R., and Snyder, F. Treatment of intractable narcolepsy with a monoamine oxidase inhibitor. New England Journal of Medicine, 285: 987-999, 1971

SLEEP, BRAIN STATE AND MEMORY[1]

James L. McGaugh, Robert A. Jensen
and Joe L. Martinez Jr.

Department of Psychobiology
University of California, Irvine

There are several meanings of the question, "What is the function of sleep?" At one level the question concerns adaptation and evolution. Why do animals sleep? What adaptive purpose does sleep serve? How does sleep aid survival? Even these general, but simple questions may be improperly phrased. One might, on logical grounds ask, instead, "Why do we awaken?" The choice of asking about sleep no doubt reflects an unstated assumption that wakefulness does not need explaining while sleep does. However, it could be argued that sleep is the normal or primary state and that wakefulness is necessary only because animals must awaken in order to eat and reproduce. It seems more appropriate to ask what evolutionary functions are served by cyclical patterns of sleep and wakefulness.

At another level, questions concerning the functions of sleep are based on assumptions that sleep states serve some homeostatic functions. Theories postulating a restorative function of sleep are based on a homeostatic model. (e.g. Coriat, 1912) Such views guide the search for fatigue products produced by wakefulness and generally assume that sleep states act in some way to return the brain and body to an unfatigued state.

[1]*Supported by USPHS research grant MH12526 and Postdoctoral Fellowship MH05358.*

Copyright © 1979 by Academic Press, Inc.
All rights of reproduction in any form reserved.
ISBN 0-12-222340-3

Again, one might view sleep and wakefulness in another way.
Perhaps sleep states induce wakefulness which then subsides
over time with decline of the arousing conditions produced by
the sleep state. The more specific questions to be asked at
this level concern the mechanisms by which cyclical changes in
wakefulness and sleep are produced. For example, there is
extensive evidence that the contents of cerebrospinal fluid
(Pappenheimer, 1967) and brain perfusates (Drucker-Colin *et al*,
1977) differ in the various states of sleep. Further, wakefulness and sleep can be induced by administering such perfusates
into the brains of recipient animals (Drucker-Colin, 1972). The
precise role that proteins and peptides play in the regulation
of cycles of sleep and wakefulness remains to be determined.
    A third type of question concerns the functions of the
neurobiological changes associated with sleep cycles and wakefulness. These changes may have functions that are unrelated
to the regulation of sleep and waking. For example, several
hormones are released during sleep (Takahashi *et al*, 1974;
Sassin, 1977). However, these hormones do not appear to be
involved in the regulation of sleep. What functions do they
serve? It might be that their effects are simply non-functional
correlates (or by-products) of more fundamental sleep mechanisms.
However, it seems more likely that hormone release and other
physiological changes associated with cycles of sleep and
wakefulness are important in regulating other physiological
processes.

BRAIN STATE AND MEMORY

    There is considerable speculation and some evidence suggest-
ing that sleep affects memory -- or more generally, that states
of sleep and wakefulness have different effects on memory.
Under some conditions, sleep can impair memory. Recent findings
indicate that, in human subjects, retention is poor if a short
period of sleep occurs just prior to learning (Ekstrand *et al*,
1977). These results suggest that processes occurring during
the early stages of sleep produce a brain state that is unfavorable for the storage of new information. It has long been
known that retention of recently-learned information is generally
best when sleep occurs after learning (Jenkins and Dallenbach,
1924). The sleep state might act by retarding the neural
processes underlying decay of retention by preventing the for-
getting that would otherwise occur during wakefulness if new
information is learned (retroactive interference), and/or by
affecting memory consolidation processes. There appear to be
states that are unfavorable for memory storage and states that
are optimal for memory storage. Extensive evidence indicates

that retention of newly-learned information is influenced by
brain states that occur (or are induced) shortly after learning.
Studies of retrograde amnesia and enhancement of memory in
laboratory animals indicate that retention can be altered by
numerous experimental treatments that alter brain functioning.
Effective treatments include electrical stimulation of the
brain, convulsant drugs, drugs affecting RNA and protein synthesis, drugs affecting catecholamine metabolism, and peptide
hormones (McGaugh and Herz, 1972; McGaugh et al, 1975). While
each treatment has a unique set of effects on brain functioning
a common property of the diverse effects is an alteration in
brain state. Studies of the relationship between brain state
and retention have suggested that EEG Theta activity is in
some way important for retention. A number of studies have
shown that, in rats, retention is best when EEG Theta activity
is recorded from the hippocampus and overlying cortex shortly
after training (Landfield,   ). EEG
Theta activity may reflect a brain state favorable for memory
consolidation.

Recent experiments have also shown that the modulating
influences of posttraining treatment on retention can be
attenuated by a variety of conditions. The retrograde amnesia
produced by ECS and protein synthesis inhibitors can be attenuated by a variety of stimulant drugs, including strychnine,
caffeine, pentylenetetrazol, and amphetamine as well as the
ACTH analog $ACTH_{4-10}$ if the drugs are administered shortly
after training (McGaugh, 1968;   Flood et al, 1977). The
fact that these drugs do not enhance protein synthesis suggests
that they act in some more general way to counteract the amnestic
influence of protein synthesis inhibitors. A simple interpretation of results such as these is that the treatments act by
influencing brain states such that they are more or less favorable for storing new information.

Thus, there is substantial evidence that experimentally
produced alterations in brain states modulate memory storage
processes. There is also evidence that retention of newly-
found information is modulated by states of sleep. In a series
of studies Bloch and his associates (Bloch et al, 1977) have
shown that retention is influenced by REM sleep occurring shortly
after training. Rats were trained on a simple task and REM
sleep was recorded after each daily training session. During
the early stages of training, REM sleep increased after each
training session. As learning progressed, the amount of REM
sleep decreased but increased again if the rats were taught a
new task. Acquisition was retarded if the rats were deprived
of REM sleep after each training session. Further, posttraining
electrical stimulation of the mesencephalic reticular formation
eliminated the impairing effect of posttraining REM deprivation

and also attenuated the amount of REM sleep occurring following training. Evidence from other laboratories has also indicated that deprivation of REM during the posttraining period impairs subsequent retention (e.g., Pearlman and Becker, 1973). Fishbein *et al* (1971) found that ECS administered 2 days after training produced a retention deficit in mice deprived of REM sleep during the 2 day period between the training and ECS treatment. Thus, posttrial REM sleep appears to modulate retention.

It is not clear what aspects of REM deprivation are responsible for the modulation of memory storage processes. No doubt deprivation of REM has many effects. It might be that the arousal, as seen in the EEG associated with REM sleep, is important for learning. Hormones released during REM sleep might also serve as memory storage modulators.

There is increasing evidence that memory storage processes are influenced by endogenous modulators. Retention is altered by posttraining administration of catecholamines, including epinephrine and norepinephrine, pituatary hormones, and neuropeptides as well as drugs that affect the functioning of these substances (McGaugh *et al*, 1975; Gold and McGaugh, 1977; Zornetzer, 1978; Rigter and van Riezen, 1978; Messing *et al*, 1978).

In view of this recent evidence it seems reasonable to speculate that the release of these "endogenous modulators" varies with different stages of sleep and wakefulness. Such patterns have already been described for some hormones. While it is known, for example, that ACTH release varies with the basic circadian rhythm, the pattern of secretion is not closely related to the sleep-waking cycle. Most research concerned with sleep and hormones appears to be focused on the possible role of hormones in the regulation of sleep and waking. Perhaps a more important secretion and the possible role of such variations in influencing processes involved in memory.

Viewed from this perspective, one important function of sleep seems to be the modulation of memory storage processes. Since storage processes remain susceptible to modulating influences for several hours after learning, cyclical stages of sleep and waking seem to provide a means of enhancing the retention of each day's experience. The evidence that a short period of sleep impairs retention of information learned after sleeping suggests that the early stages of sleep may be associated with a brain state that is unfavorable for memory storage (Ekstrand *et al*, 1977). Such a process would thus act to favor the retention of information learned prior to sleeping. From this point of view the normal human sleep-waking cycle seems well suited to favor retention.

In summary, there is much evidence connected with the general view that neurobiological correlates of sleep states modulate memory storage processes. Further study of the specific correlates responsible for the modulating influences as well as the mechanisms of action should contribute significantly to our understanding of sleep, brain states, and memory.

REFERENCES

Bloch, V., Hennevin, E., and Leconte, P. Interaction between post-trial reticular stimulation and subsequent paradoxical sleep in memory consolidation processes. pp 255-272 in Drucker-Colin, R. R., and McGaugh, J. L. (Eds), *Neurobiology of Sleep and Memory*. Academic Press, New York, 1977.

Coriat, I. H. The nature of sleep. *J. Abnormal Psych.* 1912, *6*, 329-367.

Drucker-Colin, R. R. Transmisión neurohumoral en sueno: efecto de un perfusado de la formación reticular, *Res. 15º Congr. Nac Cienc. fisiol.* 1972, pp 8 San cristobal las Casas, Chis. México

Drucker-Colin, R. R., Spanis, C. W., and Rojas-Ramírez. Investigation of the role of proteins in REM sleep. pp 303-319 in Drucker-Colin, R. R., and McGaugh, J. L. (Eds), *Neurobiology of Sleep and Memory*. Academic Press, New York, 1977.

Ekstrand, B. R., Barrett, T. R., West, J. N., and Maier, W. G. The effect of sleep on human long-term memory. pp 419-438 in Drucker-Colin, R. R., and McGaugh, J. L. (Eds), *Neurobiology of Sleep and Memory*. Academic Press, New York, 1977.

Fishbein, W., McGaugh, J. L., and Swarz, J. R. Retrograde amnesia: electroconvulsive shock after termination of rapid eye movement sleept deprivation. *Science,* 1971, *182*, 80-82.

Flood, James F., Jarvik, Murray E., Bennett, Edward L., Orme, Ann E., and Rosenzweig, Mark R. The effects of stimulants, depressants, and protein synthesis inhibition on retention. *Beh. Biol.,* 1977, *20*, 168-183.

Gold, P. E., and McGaugh, J. L. Hormones, and Memory. pp 127-143 in Miller, L. H., Sandman, C. A., and Kastin, A. J. (Eds), *Neuropeptide influences on the Brain and Behavior*. Raven Press, New York, 1977.

Jenkins, J. B., and Dallenbach, K. M., Oblivescence during sleep and waking. *Am. J. Psychol.*, 1924, *35*, 605-612.

Landsfield, P. W. Synchronous EEG rhythms: their nature and their possible functions in memory information transmission and behavior. pp 389-424 in Gispen, W. H. (Ed), *Molecular and Functional Neurobiology.* Elsevier, Amsterdam, 1976.

McGaugh, J. L. Drug effects on Learning and Memory. pp 891-904 in Efron, D. H., Cole, J. O., Levine, J., and Wittenborn, J. R. (Eds). *Psychopharmacology, a Review of Progress,* 1957-1967. U.S. Govt. Printing Office, Washington, D. C. 1968.

McGaugh, J. L., Gold, P. E., van Buskirk, R. B., and Haycock, J. W. Modulating influences of hormones and catecholamines on memory storage processes, pp 151-162. In *Hormones, Homeostasis and the Brain,* Vol. 42 of Progress in Brain Research. Gispen, W. H., van Wimersma-Greidanus, Tj. B., Bohus, B., and de Wied, D. (Eds). Elsevier, Amsterdam, 1975.

McGaugh, J. L., and Herz, M. J. *Memory Consolidation,* Albion Publishing Co., San Francisco, 1972.

Messing, R. B., Jensen, R. A., Martinez, Jr., J. L., Basquez, B. J. Soumireau-Mourat, B., and McGaugh, J. L. Naloxone enhancement and morphine impairment of memory. *Proc. of VII International Congress for Pharmacology,* 1978, p 560.

Pappenheimer, J. R., Miller, J. B., and Goodrich, C. A. Sleep promoting effects of cerebrospinal fluid from sleep-deprived goats. *Proc. Nat. Acad. Sci.* (Wash.) 1967, *58*, 513-517.

Pearlman, C., and Becker, M. B. Brief posttrial REM sleep deprivation impairs discrimination learning in rats. *Physiological Psychology,* 1973, *1*, 373-376.

Rigter, H., and van Riezen, H. Hormones and Memory. pp 677-689 in Lipton, M. A., DiMascio, A., and Killiam, K. F. (Eds), *Pharmacology, a Generation of Progress,* Raven Press, New York, 1978.

Sassin, J. F. Sleep-related hormones. pp 361-372 in Drucker-Colin, R. R., and McGaugh, J. L. (Eds), *Neurobiology of Sleep and Memory.* Academic Press, New York, 1977.

Takahashi, K., Takahashi, Y., Takahashi,S., and Honda, Y. Growth hormone and cortisol secretion during nocturnal sleep in narcoleptics and in dogs. In N. Hadotoni (Ed), *Psychoneuroendocrinology,* B. Karger, Basel, Basel, Switzerland, 1974.

Zornetzer, S. F. Neurotransmitter modulation and memory: A new neuropharmacological phrenology? pp 637-649 in Lipton, M. A., DiMascio, A., and Killiam, K. F. (Eds), *Pharmacology, a Generation of Progress,* Raven Press, New York, 1978.